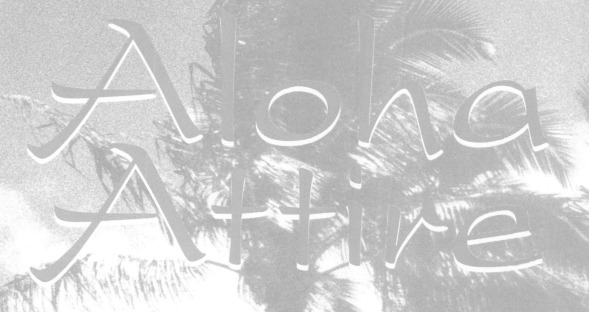

Aloha Attire

Hawaiian Dress in the Twentieth Century

Linda B. Arthur

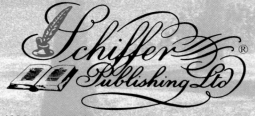

Schiffer Publishing Ltd

4880 Lower Valley Road, Atglen, PA 19310 USA

Dedication

To: Janis Okino, Genvieve Kekuninahinaokalani Bauckham, Napua F. Visser, Shanti Kamaua Haruko Miguel, Ying Yng Lee, Tamara Sullivan, Keri Murakami, and Marla Nakata.

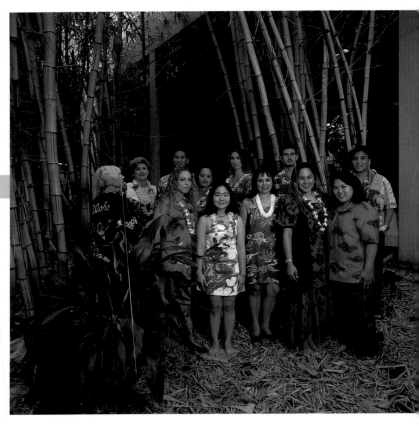

Back row, left to right: Linda B. Arthur, Douglas James Martin, Caprice Keolani Ribuca, Napua F. Visser, Clinton A. Lee and Dylan-Joshua Cabalo. Front row, left to right: Marcia Morgado, Melissa Kananiokahonoua Carlson, Janis Okino, Genvieve Kekuninahinaokalani Bauckham, Shanti Kamaua Haruko Miguel and Michelle Kam.

ISBN: 0-7643-1015-1

Cover & Book Design by Anne Davidsen
Typeset in Seagull Heavy/Aldine721

Printed in China
1 2 3 4

Published by Schiffer Publishing Ltd.
4880 Lower Valley Road
Atglen, PA 19310
Phone: (610) 593-1777; Fax: (610) 593-2002
e-mail: schifferbk@aol.com
Please visit our website catalog at
www.schifferbooks.com
or write for a free printed catalog.
This book may be purchased from the publisher.
Please include $3.95 for shipping.

In Europe, Schiffer books are distributed by
Bushwood Books
6 Marksbury Avenue
Kew Gardens
Surrey TW9 4JF England
Phone: 44 (0)208 392-8585; Fax: 44 (0)208 392-9876
e-mail: bushwd@aol.com

Please try your bookstore first.

We are interested in hearing from authors with book ideas on related subjects.

Contents

Acknowledgments

A work of this magnitude is not done by one person alone; a team of passionate historians, collectors, students, colleagues and friends helped tremendously in the development of this book. Colleagues at the University of Hawai'i in the College of Tropical Agriculture and Human Resources who provided support of all types include Drs. Charles and Barbara Laughlin, Dr. Wayne Iwaoka, Dr. Barbara Harger, Ms. Marcia Morgado, and Ms. Diane Chung. Several collectors of Hawaiian apparel provided invaluable assistance, especially with regard to the ever-changing values of Hawaiiana; my thanks go to Richard Smith, of Fullerton, CA, Camille Shaheen-Tunberg, of Venice, CA, and John Cook of Island Treasures Antiques in Honolulu, whose passion for aloha attire is contagious.

Conducting historical research is like taking a long drive on windy mountain roads; the path was made clear with the help of historian DeSoto Brown, Archivist for the Bishop Museum, who sees Hawaiian history through nineteenth and twentieth century camera lenses. Similarly, the road through the history of our garment industry was made more accessible by Ms. Carol Pregill, Executive Director of the Hawai'i Fashion Industry Association, who suggested people to interview. Several garment manufacturers, notably Mr. Alfred Shaheen, Mr. Mort Feldman and Mr. Josh Feldman, provided an enormous amount of historical data when they allowed me into their company's archives.

This book, however, could not have even been attempted without the tireless help of my devoted students. The photo sessions that produced the pictures seen here took a team of five to eight students working alongside me for thousands of hours. My most heartfelt thanks go to my talented assistants, Janis Okino, Genvieve Kekuninahinaokalani Bauckham, Napua F. Visser, Shanti Kamaua Haruko Miguel, Ying Yng Lee, Tamara Sullivan, Keri Murakami, and Marla Nakata. It is to these talented young women that this book is dedicated.

Millions of people who've never been to Hawaii know what "Hawaiian Shirts" are. They're worn, sold and even manufactured in countries all over the world. Many of these present-day shirts owe their designs to those created in Hawai`i forty to fifty years ago. But even the people who collect the vintage garments themselves probably know very little of their fascinating, complicated history. So many years later, the facts are very difficult to find, and in many cases have never been written down before.

Aloha Attire: Hawaiian Dress In The Twentieth Century is a major step towards setting the story straight. Furthermore, it goes beyond just the famous shirts to describe in more detail Hawaiian fashions in general, including those for women; and how an industry created in one small location influenced fashions worldwide. Since none of us are able to travel back in time to go shopping for the original clothing itself (at the original prices – unfortunately), reading about it will be the best we can do. So here's the book to tell you about aloha wear.

DeSoto Brown
Collector, author, archivist

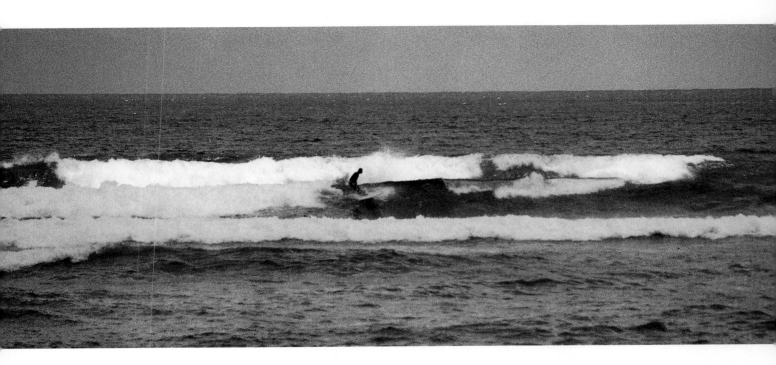

1. Aloha Attire
An Introduction

I spent several months in the Sandwich Islands [in 1867] and if I could have my way about it, I would go back there and remain the rest of my days. It is paradise ... The climate is simply delicious — never cold at sea level and never really too warm ... the green tone of a forest washes over the edges of a broad bar of orange trees that embrace the mountain like a belt, and it's so deep and dark a green that distance makes it black. ... You will note the kinds and colors of all the vegetation, just with a glance of the eye (Mark Twain, 1873).[1]

Mark Twain was just one of the many celebrated visitors who referred to Hawai`i as a paradise. Most people have been thrilled by the wonderful climate and the riot of color found in the flowering trees and other vegetation of Hawai`i. These things have not changed since Twain's visit over a century ago. Similarly, Mark Twain described the kindness and generosity of the local inhabitants, whose way of life focused on the 'spirit of aloha.' This spirit is one that embraces and welcomes ethnic diversity. The spirit of aloha is visibly manifest in contemporary Hawaiian dress, known as 'aloha attire.'

Aloha attire is a form of dress that is distinctive, due to the vibrant floral patterns found in Hawaiian textiles, and to the unique garment styles that evolved as an adaptation to the tropical environment of Hawai`i. Aloha attire refers to four traditional garment types worn in Hawai`i; the holoku, the mu`umu`u, the holomu`u, all worn by women, and the aloha shirt worn by men. In addition, there is now an evolving style of women's aloha attire that is global in impact and is more generally termed resort wear. In Hawai`i, a multi-cultural society with no ethnic majority, aloha attire is worn as a unifying symbol connecting people with the unique tropical locale of Hawai`i. Aloha attire is regularly worn on Fridays - every Friday is Aloha Friday. Additionally, it is considered dressier than western-styled clothing, and is worn to church and other special events. Aloha attire is commonly found at rites of passage such as baby luau, graduations, weddings and funerals.

Aloha attire helps to define the residents of the Hawaiian Islands (Oahu, The Big Island (Hawai`i), Maui, Kauai, Molokai, Lanai, Ni'ihau, Kaho'olawe). The unique Hawaiian lifestyle includes the cosmopolitan culture of the people of Hawai`i. Maintaining elements of Hawaiian culture is a way of life, from eating Hawaiian foods to speaking pidgin English, to wearing aloha attire.[2]

As part of a six year project on the history of Hawaiian dress[3], this book is the result of research that included both primary sources (his-

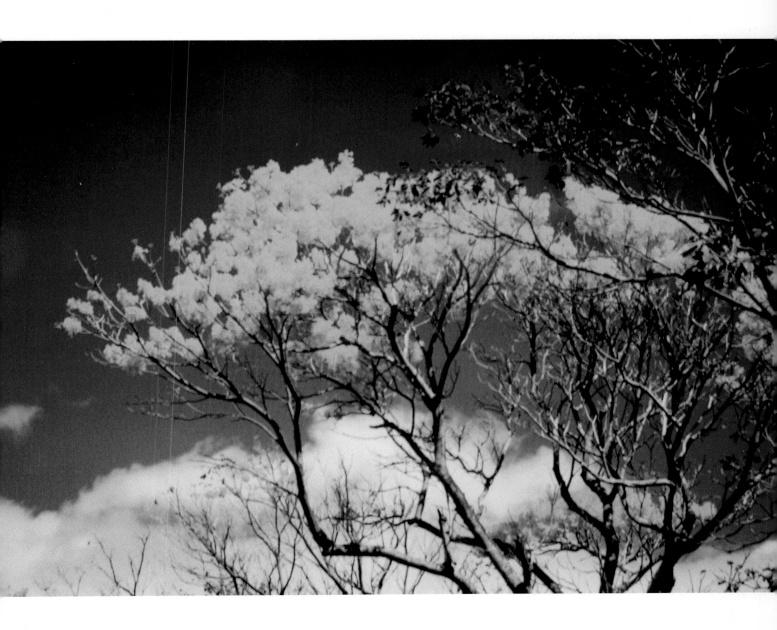

torical records, diaries, traveler's accounts, photographs, museum collections and interviews) and secondary sources (books, newspaper articles, archives of museums, collections and libraries). The importance of the primary sources, particularly the 990 photographs, 1010 garments and textile swatches studied, must be stressed as they yield greater historical accuracy.

The focus of *Aloha Attire: Hawaiian Dress In The Twentieth Century* is to present a comprehensive view of garments that were produced in, and worn by the people of Hawai`i, which is a departure from the books currently on the market. Books published on Hawaiian clothing thus far feature garments (mostly rayon aloha shirts from the late 1940s and 1950s) that have ended up in private collections from Japan to the mainland US. These books often include serious inaccuracies, especially regarding dates attributed to aloha shirts. *Aloha Attire: Hawaiian Dress In The Twentieth Century* is an attempt to present a historically accurate discussion of how people in Hawai`i have dressed in aloha attire throughout the twentieth century.

7

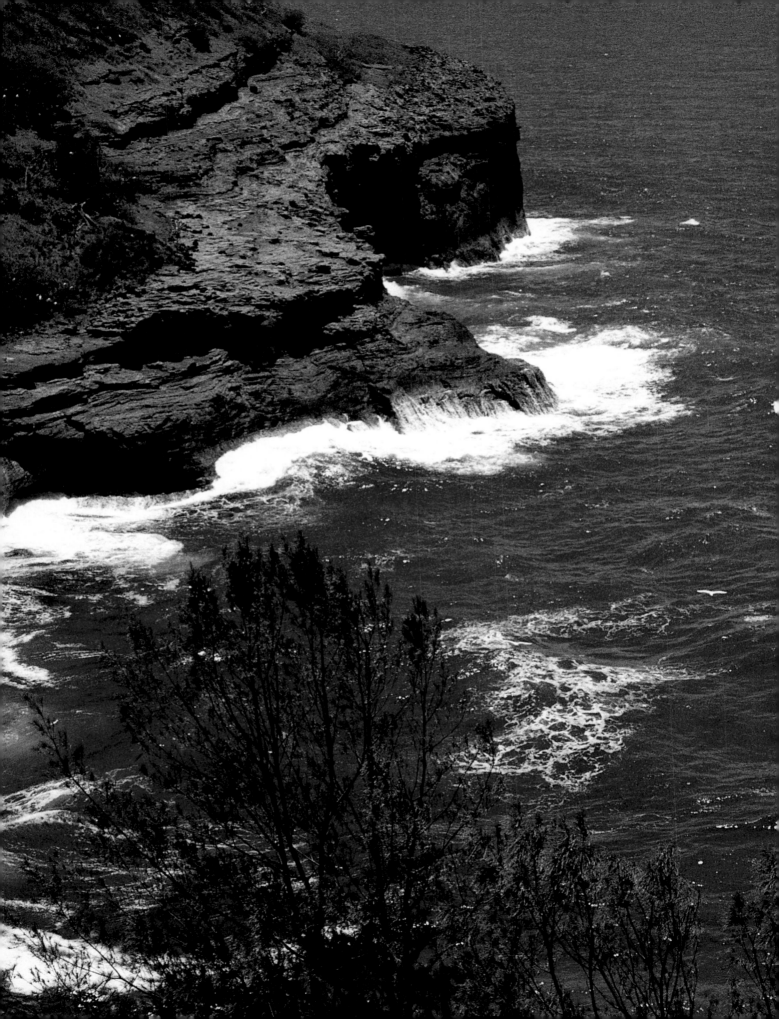

2. Hawaiian Clothing
Historical Background

During the nineteenth century, the Hawaiian kingdom was ruled by a series of kings with powerful queens at their side. Kamehameha the Great was a strong ruler who united all the islands under his control. His favorite wife, Kaahumanu, was a powerful woman who raised his son Liholiho to be King Kamehameha II. Kaahumanu was an important figure who is partly responsible for the shift from garments made of barkcloth (kapa) to clothing made of woven fabric. Within a week of meeting missionary women dressed in fabric gowns, she adopted a similar garment that became known as the holoku.

Before the arrival of permanent residents from the Western world, the indigenous Hawaiians had contact with outsiders through the sandalwood trade. This was a lucrative business for the Hawaiians, and the royalty were able to live in splendor befitting their station in life. In trade for sandalwood, the ali'i (royalty) began to amass quantities of woven fabric.

Prior to the arrival of missionaries, the standard Hawaiian costume consisted of only a brief lower body covering for both sexes. Indigenous Hawaiians made and wore kapa cloth by felting fibers from the inner bark of the paper mulberry tree. Men wore a loincloth called the malo. Ali`i might also be covered by a cape called a kihei. Women wore the pa`u, a wrapped garment of kapa that was worn in several layers, and often had applied geometric designs. The pa`u passed several times around the waist and was three to four feet long. The missionaries, upon their arrival in 1820, considered this brief costume shockingly immodest.[4] The ali`i, however, had access to men's western clothing through trade with visiting sailors and wore whatever items of western clothing they had for occasions involving interaction with westerners.[5] For Hawaiian rituals, the ali`i wore the splendid red and yellow feather capes and cloaks which had made Hawai`i famous, but they also traded feather garments to foreigners (haoles).[6]

The indigenous religion in pre-contact Hawai`i was overthrown in 1819, a year before the arrival of the Christian missionaries. However, Hawaiian society did not disintegrate because the Hawaiian monarchy was still strong and the class system provided for social structure. The religion was a complex system based on a strict division of status between the chiefly class and commoners, who provided huge quantities of food to the ali`i who feasted regularly, and whose larger size and finer clothing represented their higher social position.

One of the most rapid and visually noticeable changes was that after the arrival of missionaries, the Hawaiians began to shed their traditional kapa clothing and eventually adopted western-styled clothing. The missionary wives arrived in Hawai`i wearing dresses in the

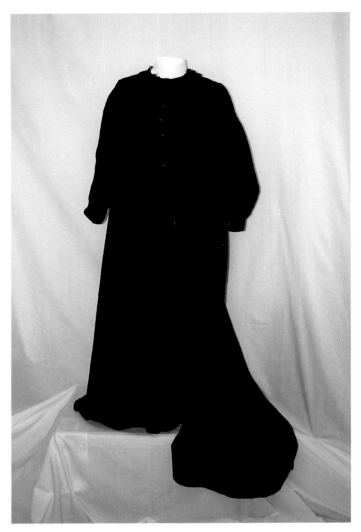

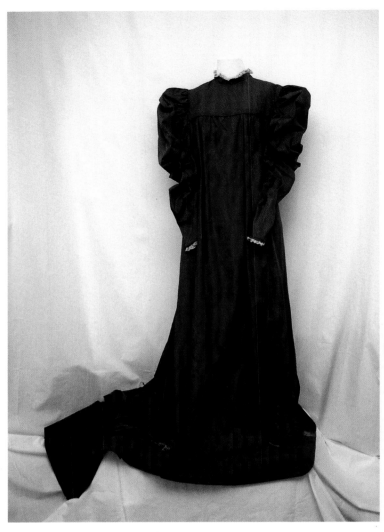

Silk jacquard holoku. Worn by member of Kaahumanu society, 1890s, 95.5.3.

Jacquard holoku, copy of 1890 silk holoku, original trims, 82.5.1.

style of 1819, with a high waist, narrow skirt and long, tight sleeves. The female ali`i were enchanted and immediately requested that similar dresses be sewn for them. The queens brought out their stores of brocades, silks, and chintz, and missionary wives were pressed into service as seamstresses.[7] In order to fit the large size of the Hawaiian women, and to adapt to the hot, humid environment, the mission ladies adapted their high-waisted style for a loose, comfortable fit.[8] They moved the waistline from underneath the bust, and replaced it with an above-the-bust yoke.[9] The end result was a basic design that was simply a full, straight skirt attached to a yoke with a high neck and tight sleeves.[10] This dress was called the holoku, and the missionaries gave the queens chemises (slips) to wear underneath; the Hawaiians called the chemises mu`umu`u.

The missionaries realized that their goal of religious conversion would not be possible without first transforming Hawaiians culturally into Americans.[11] Dress was the first issue undertaken. While the upper classes adopted western-styled clothing in the first few years after the missionaries' arrival, the commoners resisted. Naked torsos offended the missionaries, and they worked hard to coerce Hawaiians into wearing western-styled clothing. After trade with the US became brisk in the mid-nineteenth century, brightly colored fabrics were desired for the making of western-styled clothing.[12] Vibrant colors were a sign of status. Until the taboos were overthrown in 1819, the colors red and yellow were only worn by ali`i.

Hawai`i was a kingdom until the end of the nineteenth century. The Iolani Palace in Honolulu was a Victorian showplace, and the ali`i class amassed quantities of western consumer goods and clothing designed by European couturiers. First worn by the ali`i as a novel means of status display, western-styled clothing became firmly associated with upper class status in nineteenth century Hawai`i. The transition from the kapa malo for men of the commoner class to western clothing was slower than for the male chiefs who had more goods to barter. Hawaiian men traded with sailors for western clothing, and were particularly fond of the sailor's loose-fitting shirts called "frocks" that were obtained from English and American seamen. The Hawaiians transliterated the word 'frock' into 'palaka'. Frock shirts were made of heavy cotton fabric and worn loose rather than tucked into trousers. This was comfortable in Hawaii's hot, humid climate. One form of the fabric used in these early shirts was a plaid that is now known as palaka; it became a favorite fabric for men's jackets and shirts by 1900.

Late Ninteenth Century

Female ali`i wore European dress for formal occasions, and relegated the holoku to leisurewear. For the majority of Hawaiian women, the transition from the indigenous dress of kapa pa`u to the western-styled holoku was complete by the late nineteenth century. A similar transition for men from the kapa malo to western-styled pants and shirts was a bit slower. The transition for both men and women was dependent on their social status within Hawaiian culture, and their conversion to Christianity. Following its adoption by royalty, who were the first to become Christianized, the holoku and its undergarment, the mu`umu`u, were adopted by other Hawaiian women who converted to Christianity. The holoku was eventually adopted by most Hawaiian women as their economic situation allowed, by the end of the nineteenth century.[13] Due to demand for western-styled fashions, and the increased availability of woven fabric through barter, the holoku had become standard dress for Hawaiian women who worked in it, were married in it and finally, were buried in the holoku.[14]

Since American visitors had begun arriving in Hawai`i in the late nineteenth century, it is perhaps not surprising that suffragettes and other proponents of rational dress were aware of the holoku and its comfortable design. They suggested it as a possible alternative to fashionable dress (which included corsets that weighed 40 pounds). Although the short-trained cotton holoku was worn for everyday dress in Hawai`i, more importantly during the Hawaiian monarchy era, the holoku was a recognized court gown, often made of silks and satins.[15] This gown, sometimes made of lace, and with varied trims and elaborate decoration, continues today as a dominant style of formal dress in Hawai`i.

At the turn of the century, the Kamehameha dynasty came to an end. Kamehameha V died in 1872. Prince Lunalilo was selected as the new king but died a year later. David Kalakaua was chosen next: his sister Liliuokalani ruled in his absence while Kalakaua went to

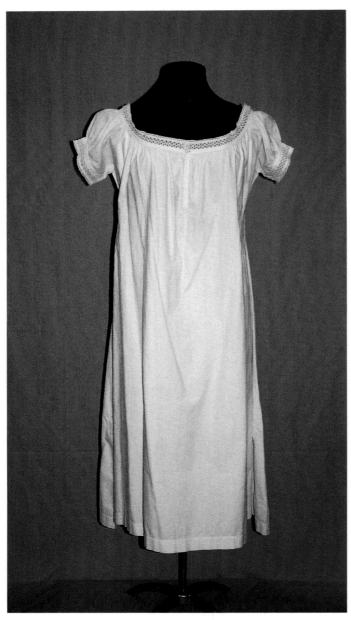

Cotton mu`umu`u, hand made lace, 1830s, 76.47.1, $700 to $999

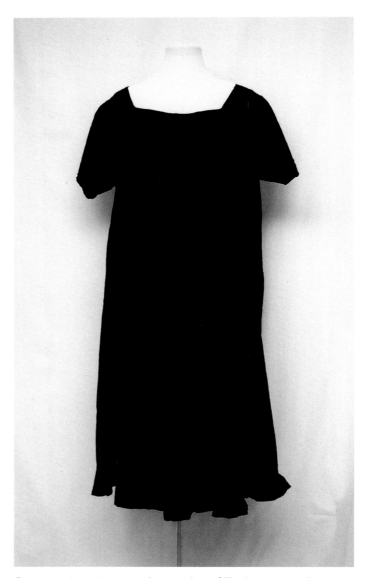

Cotton mu`umu`u, worn by member of Kaahumanu society, 1890s, 95.5.4, $1,000+

Washington to negotiate a reciprocal trade treaty. Hawaiian sugar was increasingly important in trade with the US and American money was equally important in Hawai`i. Kalakaua's attempts to increase the power of the monarchy threatened the interests of foreign businessmen. Ultimately, American businessmen managed to overthrow the Hawaiian monarchy in 1893. After the counter-revolution in 1895, Queen Liliuokalani was arrested and imprisoned in Iolani Palace.

By the end of the nineteenth century, the ethnic composition of the residents of Hawai`i had undergone a significant change. After the permanent arrival of missionaries and businessmen from America, the Hawaiian population was seriously reduced by the introduction of diseases from the Western world for which the Hawaiians had no immunity. When laborers were needed for the sugar, coffee and pineapple plantations, immigrants (primarily from Asia) were brought in, and men and women worked in the fields together. By the end of the nineteenth century, there were several ethnic groups, and the plantation system became a powerful force in Hawai`i.

Prior to the end of the nineteenth century, women made clothing for their families at home in what little spare time they had. Men without wives had to learn to sew and repair their own work clothing. While kimonos and other traditional clothing were sewn at home, male tailors and shopkeepers commercially produced custom-made men's wear, mostly in Honolulu. Immigrant women were primarily employed as seamstresses. This system of custom-made garments produced for individuals continued until 1922 when the need for work clothing led to the formation of the Hawaiian Clothing Manufacturing Company, Ltd.

3. Early Twentieth Century

Cultural Context

The early twentieth century was a study in cultural contrasts in Hawai`i. As the previous century opened, the resident population was Hawaiian. In the early twentieth century, however, the people of Hawai`i were no longer entirely Hawaiian. The population also included white businessmen and their families, who controlled the economy and the sugar and pineapple plantations. To provide laborers for the plantations, immigrant workers were brought in from Japan, China, Korea, Portugal, Okinawa and the Philippines. For many people in Hawai`i, life in the early twentieth century was hard. Plantation life was reported by some to be brutal for those on the lower end of the social scale. When Buddhist missionaries arrived in 1889, they found the workers demoralized and ill treated.[16] Over time, however, conditions improved and Hawai`i became characterized by its amicable relations between the many ethnic groups, in part because the various ethnic groups were at approximately the same social status and socialized with each other. Intermarriage between the indigenous Hawaiians and the immigrants led to the extraordinary ethnic diversity seen in Hawai`i today. As a consequence of the impact of disease on the indigenous Hawaiians, and of immigration and intermarriage, today no ethnic group is in the majority.[17]

While tourism to Hawai`i began in the nineteenth century, it increased significantly in the early twentieth century. Tourists stayed in simple hotels that only provided bed and board. Early hotels included the Moana, Haleiwa, and Alexander Young, however, the first resort hotel, the Royal Hawaiian Hotel, was built in 1927 and started a new era of tourism in Waikiki in which the tourists were offered numerous activities to enhance their travel experiences. As the fame of this hotel grew, and its reputation was known worldwide, going to Hawai`i became the vogue for the upper classes.[18]

Fabric and Clothing Production

In the early twentieth century, kapa was no longer produced as woven fabric was readily available. Printed cottons with Asian motifs were used most commonly in addition to Japanese resist-dyed ikats known as yukata cloth. These cottons were used for both western-styled clothing and kimono. Additionally, both raw silk and finely woven silks were also imported from Japan. Cottons, particularly calico and small figured cotton prints, were favorite fabrics imported from the mainland US. Kimono from Japan, as well as cheong sam and coolie outfits from China were seen in

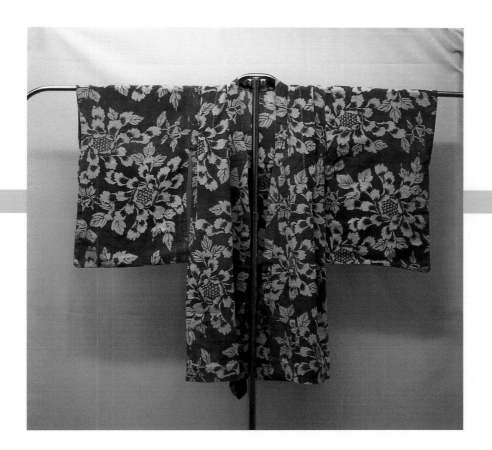

Hawai`i until the 1930s.

Women's wear was primarily produced at home in the beginning of the twentieth century, following the pattern set in the previous century. However, the influx of tailors, kimono makers and custom shirt manufacturers during the early twentieth century began the move of clothing production out of the home and into the shop. At the same time, ready made clothing (especially work clothing) was being imported into the Territory of Hawai`i from America, Asia and Europe. By 1922, the two major retailers in Honolulu, Watumull's East India Store (now Watumull's) and what became known as Liberty House (by 1929) were advertising the importation of fine clothing. Numerous ads noted fabrics for sale, indicating that most of the clothing produced in this time period was done by home sewers who provided for their own families.[19]

While most clothing was made at home, production of clothing by custom tailors, like Musa-Shiya the Shirtmaker, began producing men's western-styled shirts as well as kimono, happi coats and other Asian-styled garments. Almost all of the garments produced in the 1920s were made of silk or cotton. Hats were necessary for protection from the sun; they were made of woven lauhala and to the trained eye, could indicate what type of work the wearer performed.

In 1922, two clothing factories opened, both to produce work clothing. The Union Supply Company produced uniforms for the military as well as work pants and overalls for local workers. The Hawai`i Clothing Manufacturing Company produced work clothes for the plantation workers, as well as its trademark Sailor Moku, denim bell-bottom trousers with a full fall front with two sets of vertical buttons. These resembled sailor pants. Especially worn for casual wear, sailor moku were teamed up with palaka shirts and cotton print shirts with simple Asian designs.[20]

Women's Attire

The overthrow of the Hawaiian Kingdom in 1893 (at the hands of American businessmen) was a painful event for Hawaiians. The islands were being Americanized in both business and politics and no where was the acculturation process more visible than with clothing. Immigrant women wore clothing they brought with them from their native countries and continued to wear that traditional dress for both casual wear and for weddings. They also began to wear what the Japanese immigrant women called kanakagi, or Hawaiian wear in the early twentieth century[21]. What they meant by this term was the holoku that was the main style of dress worn by Hawaiian and immigrant women in the Islands. In addition, western fashion was being imported and was increasingly worn in Hawai`i.

The first decade of the twentieth century produced a style of holoku which has become classic; these holoku have been memorialized in paintings and have enjoyed a revival in the 1980s and 1990s. From 1900 through 1920, the short-trained holoku was the standard dress for women outside the home. The holoku continued to be worn with little significant change from the turn of the century except that white was the predominant color and more detail was added, such as ruffles and tatting. Because of these design details, the holoku was said to resemble the European tea gown; it was also referred to as "lingerie gown" due to its comfort. In 1907, the holoku was described as the "Hawaiian modification of the European tea gown."[22] Before the 1920s, holoku was made in cottons such as muslin, batiste and dimity, and had a straighter silhouette than previously. Trains lengthened, and the use of lace, eyelet, pin tucks and ruffles at the sleeves, yokes and hems increased significantly. White holoku dominated the Hawaiian fashion scene. Nonetheless, black holoku continued to be favored by many Hawaiian women, especially members of the Kaahumanu Society, who dressed in black to show allegiance to Queen Kaahumanu (favorite wife of King Kamehameha), the overthrown Hawaiian monarchy, and its last regent, Queen Liliuokalani.

The mu`umu`u was still worn underneath the holoku as an undergarment, or worn as a housedress or for swimming. The mu`umu`u was not considered fit for public view until the 1940s. It was a loose garment, with short sleeves and worn knee-length or longer. The fabric for mu`umu`u was generally in solid colored cotton.

The 1920s ushered in some changes for holoku design, and led to two versions of the holoku, based on fit. While the loose, long-sleeved lingerie style holoku remained a favorite style especially for more conservative women, a second style, the fitted holoku, became the more fashionable style. Using darts and princess lines, the holoku was fitted very closely to the body. The result was a simple tubular style. Necklines were lowered, trains lengthened and sleeves were shortened or eliminated altogether.

The development of a truly fitted holoku during the 1920s was countered with a resurgence of interest in the traditionally loose holoku. Again, the two styles coexisted comfortably in Hawai`i. Traditional Hawaiian women began re-creating the holoku from the mid-nineteenth century. While the fitted holoku continued to be fashionable,

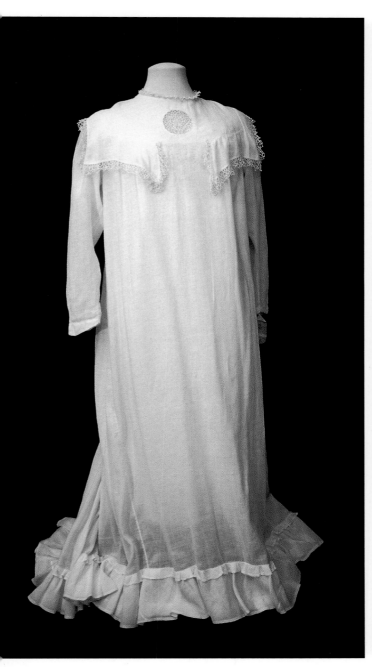

Cotton dobby weave holoku, hand made tatting trim, 1910s, 75.5.16, $1,000+

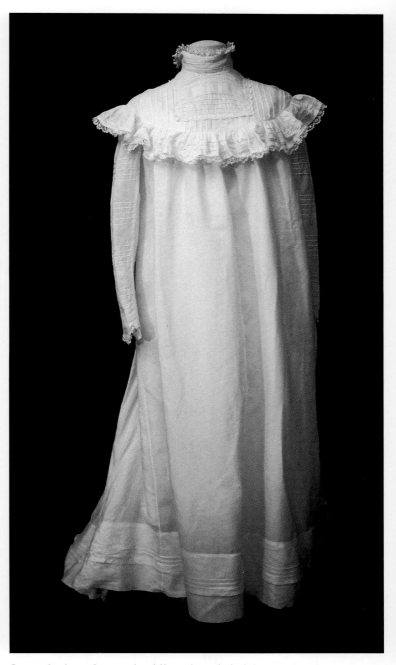

Cotton batiste, short-trained lingerie style holoku, 1910s, 93.1.1, $1,000+

the traditional style reminiscent of the missionary period re-emerged. Reverence for Hawaiian history was seen when women began copying the old family holoku, but adding contemporary features. The holoku and Hawaiian heritage are celebrated annually in the Holoku Ball, begun by the Hawaiian Civic Club in 1923.

Work clothing for women who worked on the plantation was an amalgamation of the ethnic styles brought into the Islands by the immigrants. Items of dress were adopted to suit the function of such labor. Heavy aprons, dirndl skirts, long-sleeved blouses and protective gear for arms and legs were made of a variety of cotton fabrics. Jackets were often made of a Japanese cotton called kasuri, and other garments were made of denim, called ahina in Hawai`i (ahina means blue dye).[23]

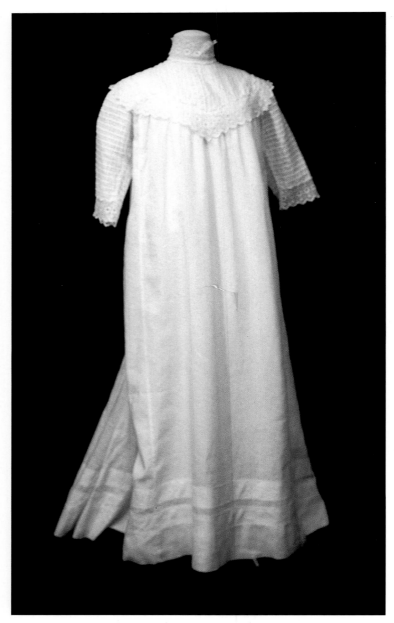

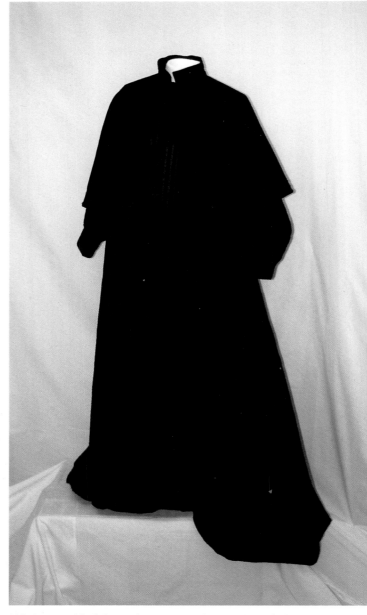

Cotton batiste, lingerie style holoku, 1910s, 93.1.3, $1,000+

Silk jacquard holoku and cape, worn by member of Kaahamanu society , 1890s, 95.5.3c, $1,000+

Men's Wear

By the turn of the century, most men were working on the plantations and wore a variety of garments. Immigrants of both sexes wore clothing they brought with them from their native countries and continued to wear that traditional dress for both casual wear and for weddings.

For work, however, it did not take long for plantation workers to see the benefits of wearing clothing made of denim. In addition to shirts and pants, denim was also used for long-sleeved work jackets, especially those worn by Japanese immigrants. The early twentieth century saw a huge variety of clothing worn by the multi-ethnic population. Denim was the staple fabric of plantation life, and was used to make pants, shirts, jackets, raincoats, skirts and aprons worn by plantation workers.

18

Palaka

The fabric known as palaka is a heavy cotton cloth woven in a white and dark blue plaid design and was in use in Hawai`i by 1900. In the nineteenth century, sailors landing on the Islands wore loose fitting, long-sleeved upper garments called frocks. The Hawaiians transliterated the word "frock" into "palaka" as they did the name "Frank" into "Palani" (In Hawaiian, there are vowels between consonants and words ending with vowels. "F" becomes ".P", and "R" becomes "L"). The woven cotton plaid design became popular and the word palaka became descriptive of the design rather than the garment itself. By the end of the nineteenth century, as immigrants came to Hawai`i and worked in the fields and mills, the use of palaka spread because of its durability, coolness, and design. The palaka shirt and palaka jacket were garments commonly worn by plantation workers of Portuguese and Hawaiian ancestry. The earliest documentation of palaka shirts and jackets occurs in pictures from 1895 to 1900. Palaka jackets became popular for plantation workers of all ethnicities by the 1920s.[24]

An Okinawan immigrant, Zempan Arakawa, saw a need for someone not only to repair field workers' clothing but to sew work clothes. He bought a foot pedal sewing machine, taught himself pattern making, and soon expanded his fledgling business by hiring housewives to do piecework while he continued working in the fields. Business flourished. After opening a tailor shop, he added general merchandise, a taxi service and hotel. Arakawa's Plantation Department Store began supplying work clothes and other needs of the plantation workers in 1909. Palaka work shirts were an important staple item.[25] Palaka, indigenous to Hawaii's workers over the years, has became a culturally significant item that has transcended ethnic differences. By 1930, palaka had become closely identified with the local population.[26]

Hawaiian men had adopted western clothing by this time. A loose, heavy cotton work shirt worn by California sailors, called the "Thousand Mile Shirt" was worn outside the trousers; it found its way to Hawai`i via sailing ships and was adopted first by Chinese laborers.[27] When this sturdy shirt was made of palaka fabric, the shirt was renamed the palaka shirt which was mass-produced for plantation laborers in the 1920s. Also in the Islands at this time was the Filipino man's shirt called the barong tagalog- a sheer, cool long-sleeved shirt worn loose over trousers. Add to this the Chinese, Japanese and Haole custom tailors in the Islands prior to the 1930s and the stage was set for all these multi-ethnic forces to blend together and create what would become the aloha shirt.

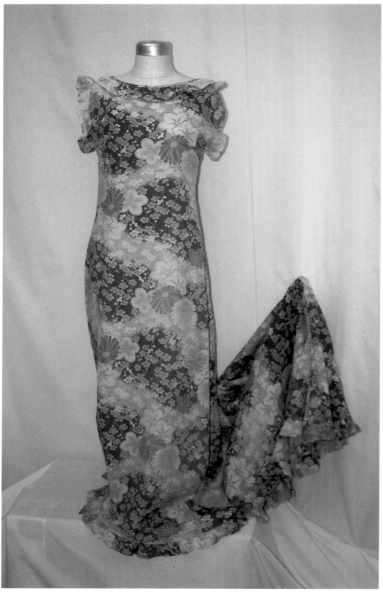

Cotton voile Japanese print holoku, 1920s, 98.2.3, $700 to $999

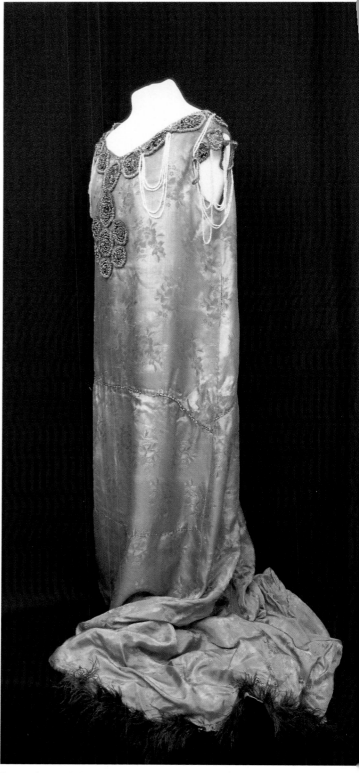

Rayon brocade holoku. Said to have been worn by Queen Lilioukalani (unsubstantiated), 1920s, 94.4.1, Courtesy of the Los Angeles County Museum of Art. $1,000+

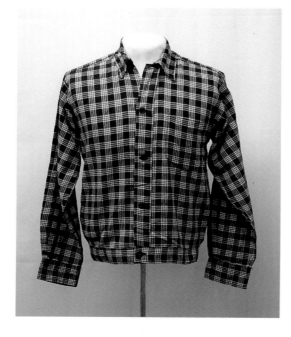

Cotton plaid palaka jacket in 1920s style. Courtesy of Barbara Kawakami, $300 to $699

4. The 1930s Through Wartime 1940s

Proto- Hawaiian Design

Cultural Context

The 1930s through the end of World War II was a period of transition in Hawaiian textile design. The transition resulted from both the availability of imported goods (primarily from Asia) to a changing sense of identity of the population. The ethic mix, which had begun with the importation of laborers in the previous century, had begun to stabilize through both necessity and intermarriage. The different ethnic groups began to come together to re-define what it meant to be Hawaiian, based on culture and a sense of place, rather than genealogy. This sense of cooperation came out of the necessity of living under the plantation's oppressive conditions. The plantation economy dominated Hawai`i until after World War II and the ramifications of this economic system permeated life on the Islands. The class differences that resulted from the plantation economy were also manifested in clothing. There was an enormous disparity between the upper class (primarily composed of white businessmen and their families, as well as kama'aina families – the descendants of the early white settlers) and the lower classes. In terms of population, the vast majority of the people in Hawai`i were on the lower end of the socio-economic scale. Native Hawaiians were not privy to the economic growth of the times, nor were the plantation workers (who were primarily immigrants) and their descendants.

The 1930s saw the beginning of tourism as a major Hawaiian industry, and coupled with the increase of US military personnel stationed in Hawai`i led to a global awareness of Hawai`i. By the 1930s the promotional efforts of the Hawai`i Tourist Bureau, already in existence for thirty years, were focused on promoting the Territory as a romantic tourist destination. Color and Hawai`i go together. The intense color found in the Islands' fish and flowers was hyped in the promotional literature that was already abundant by the 1930s. Flowers were praised continually, such as "the most ethereal of all the island flowers is the delicate moon-worshipping cereus, which blooms only at night." Don Blanding wrote of the beauty of Hawaiian skies in *Hula Moons:* "The sun, grand master of ceremonies, retired behind a curtain of sultry colors, leaving the scene set with towering trade clouds piled like white phantoms of temples." The Tourist Bureau's ads such as the one below capitalized on that exoticism: "Hawai`i nights! Hawaiian moon. And it's not a moon to be trifled with. It is potent ... bewitching ... (just to look is an adventure)."[28] The stage was thus set for the depiction of Hawaiian flora and fauna on the textiles produced in the next decade.

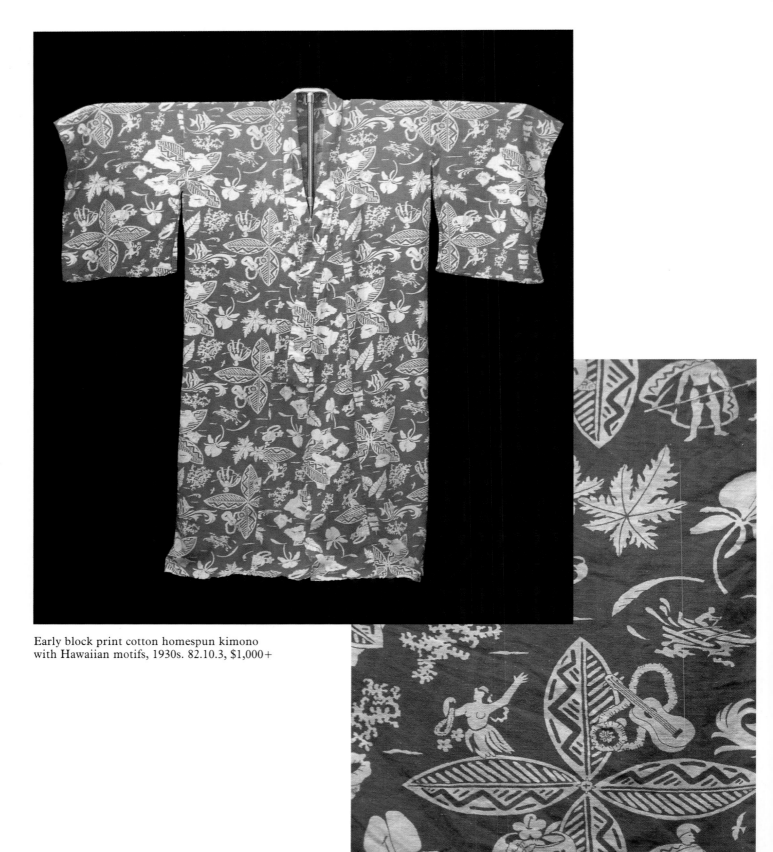

Early block print cotton homespun kimono
with Hawaiian motifs, 1930s. 82.10.3, $1,000+

Block print fabric, Hawaiian motifs, 1930s.

22

Fabrics

The many errors found in other books on Hawaiian shirts can be attributed to a misunderstanding of the textiles found in Hawai`i in the 1930s. As a clothing manufacturer who began production in the 1940s noted, with regard to the existing books on aloha shirts, "There is so much misinformation out there and people who take the posture of an expert when they really don't know the evolution of Hawaiian designs and the aloha shirt."[29] To understand the development of the aloha shirt, one must first understand what textiles were in use in Hawai`i prior to the end of World War II. Plain cotton broadcloth was, by far, the dominant fabric for all garments, from the holoku, mu`umu`u and kimono, to the aloha shirt. These were done in light-weight cotton fabrics, such as Japanese yukata cloth, with figures and flora on a blue or black background the most popular.[30] Silk, kabe crepe and challis (usually a fine wool) were used for dressier shirts or women's garments. Undergarments were made either of fine silk, for the upper classes, or lightweight rayon, for the lower classes. This rayon was much like today's nylon tricot, often found in underwear. It was unsuitable for printing and did not have the strength and texture necessary to retain vivid color. (It was not until the 1940s that a heavier rayon was developed and could hold color.) The early aloha shirts were made with kimono fabrics of silk or kabe crepe, or of simple cotton broadcloth two color prints. The design motifs on the early 1930s aloha shirts were uniformly Asian and were generally roller printed, then imported into Hawai`i. During the War, due to the restrictions on trade, fabrics in Hawai`i were frequently screen printed.

Raw silk was occasionally used for garments, and along with a heavy cotton, also used for draperies in the 1930s. The role of fabrics for interior designs is important to consider as the original Hawaiian tropical prints were designed for draperies and upholstery, not garments. Consequently, claims found in other books that date Hawaiian tropical prints on rayon garments to the 1930s are inaccurate.[31]

Elsie Das, a designer commissioned by Watumull's East India Store in 1936, created a series of fifteen Hawaiian designs on raw silk that became her trademark. What is often missed by previous authors who have written about Hawaiian design is that Elsie Das' original designs were made for interior decoration, not for clothing.[32]

Pictures at the Bishop Museum show people (even celebrities like Bing Crosby) in Hawai`i wearing cotton shirts with Japanese motifs in the 1930s. By 1937, some long-sleeved shirts were made of drapery fabric with tropical designs in very large scale. At about the same time, two color broadcloth prints appear with Hawaiian words; these designs resemble stickers put on luggage during this time period (1934-1935). The earliest pictures of prints with Hawaiian floral motifs thus far are from 1938 and 1939; it seems clear that Hawaiian prints made in cottons began to be seen on apparel around 1938. While a few rayon garments were produced in the late 1930s, the fabric was of inferior quality and did not hold color well. Virtually all of the vintage garments still in existence made of Hawaiian prints on rayon were produced **after** World War II.

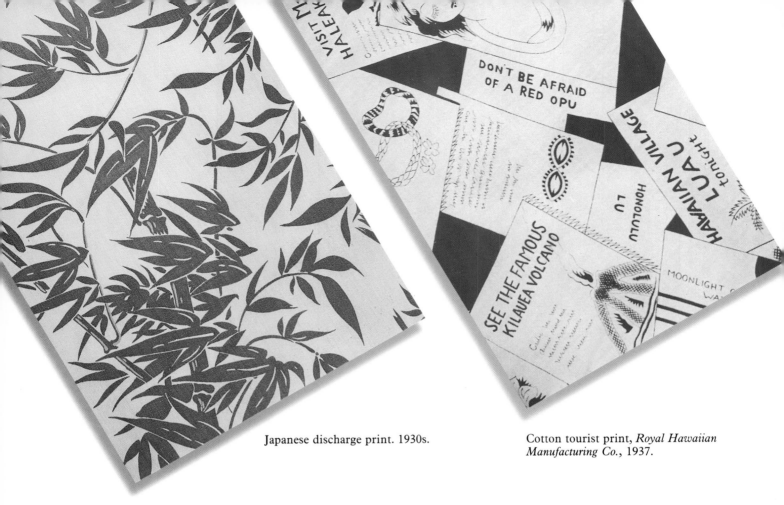

Japanese discharge print. 1930s.

Cotton tourist print, *Royal Hawaiian Manufacturing Co.*, 1937.

Shipping between Hawai`i and the US was curtailed during World War II and this set the stage for an industry which could neither import nor export garments. Fabrics had to be printed locally. Due to the scarcity of imported western-styled clothing, aloha attire became more popular on the Islands for the local population. For some time, tourists and military personnel had readily adopted aloha shirts, but due to a lack of other options, the local Islanders began to accept them as well. Locally produced fabrics in Hawaiian prints were sewn into women's wear as well. The mu`umu`u was no longer seen as a housedress once it was made of Hawaiian prints. Similarly, holoku were produced in Hawaiian prints during the War and post-War years.

Clothing Production

Women's clothing and kimono continued to be produced at home, or were imported, throughout the 1930s. The decade began with the mass production of work clothing, and ended up with the industry's focus primarily on sportswear (which dominates today, at the end of the twentieth century). In the early 1930s, most of the clothing manufactured in Hawai`i was work clothing, although casual clothing, such as sailor moku pants, and even sailor moku swimsuits began to dominate by the mid 1930s. It was in 1936 that two major garment manufacturers, Kamehameha and Branfleet set up factories in order to produce sportswear. Both were founded by men with American fashion industry experience and both targeted tourists in Hawai`i and consumers on the US mainland as major outlets for Hawaiian garment production. The clothing needs of Hawaiian residents were put to the background, due to economics. Hawai`i was still a plantation economy, with the bulk of its population primarily in the lower classes. Only the

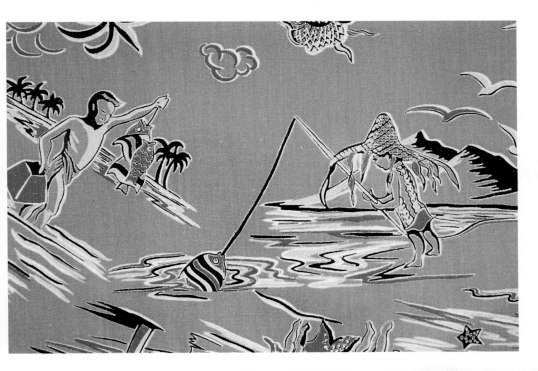

Cotton print with keiki (children) fishing, early aloha shirt, 1930s.

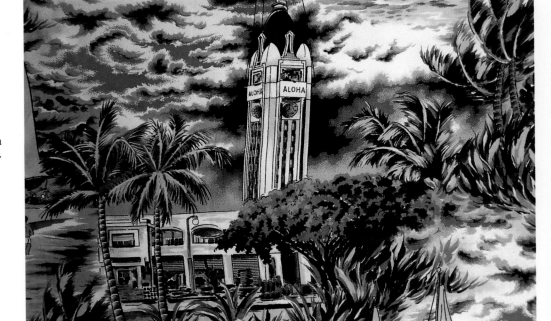

Kabe crepe from Japan, Aloha Tower design.

upper classes could afford clothing for leisure activities: "It was the Depression, then, and still Plantation days. I didn't know anyone who could afford aloha shirts when they first came out, and my family wasn't poor like most," said a Chinese-American gentleman.[33]

Kamehameha was the dominant garment manufacturer of the 1930s, but its market relied on the mainland US and tourists. Kamehameha's famous anthurium print shirt was originally done in the late '30s on raw silk. Recalled Mr. Herb Briner, "It was the beginning and almost the end of Kamehameha ... because of the unstable quality of the imported fabric." Dyes faded on raw silk so Briner came up with an alternative. They found a certain type of cotton grown in Peru that had practically no shrinkage; the cotton was shipped to Japan for printing and then back to Kamehameha in Hawai`i where it was sewn into garments. The switch to more dependable yardage turned out to be the successful launching of prints for Island sportswear.[34]

25

1936 and 1937 were significant years, marking the beginning of mass-produced apparel in Hawai`i. Herbert Briner started Kamehameha Garment Company in 1936. He came to the islands on a mission for the May Co. to find out why dyes faded in raw silk. He began to work for the Oahu Garment Company but soon bought out the company and changed its name to Kamehameha. Originally a small plant in Honolulu that manufactured men's raw silk shirts, Kamehameha grew and the company was relocated to the Big Island in Hilo where they had a ready pool of trained women as seamstresses. Briner served as president and handled local sales, while Millie Briner was designer for the firm. In the early years, Kamehameha's fabrics were designed in Hawai`i, printed in California, and manufactured into shirts in Hawai`i. During the Christmas season of 1936, a shipping strike caused the fabric to be stranded in California and the finished garments in Hawai`i. The companies tried to sell the garments locally, but people in Hawai`i didn't buy the shirts so Briner began exporting to America, Europe, New Zealand and Australia. Only five percent of their garments were sold locally. In 1939 Kamehameha produced "23 exclusive print designs ... all of the cottons being printed on the mainland."[35]

Branfleet, (later renamed Kahala Sportswear) was also founded in 1936 by George Brangier and Nat Norfleet. Today, like Kamehameha, Kahala is one of the oldest and largest firms on the islands. Along with Kamehameha, the company began by selling aloha shirts made of kabe crepes, in Asian designs. They also supplied sportswear to the mainland on a large scale. By 1939, the most popular prints were still quite subtle with small motifs and little color contrast. The best selling designs were a shell tapa of Polynesian inspiration and an aloha tapa. Only upon a closer look could one see the word "aloha" designed into the pattern. These basic designs with slight modifications were used through the end of World War II.[36] Branfleet's company trademark was the pineapple tweed. The fabric looked like rough linen; it was a durable fabric constructed into plain, solid colored shirts with long sleeves and open collars. These shirts were also referred to as jackets. The only decoration was the Royal Hawaiian crest with the motto: "The life of the land is perpetuated in righteousness." In 1939 the company produced a line of Duke Kahanamoku swimwear using solid colored pineapple tweed, but had to be curtailed due to shortages of materials during World War II. This was the first of three different licensing agreements using Duke's name and no rayon print shirts were produced with the Duke Kahanamoku label until after 1950.[37]

Tourism continued to grow, and that unique demand led to the development of the Royal Hawaiian Manufacturing Company, founded in 1937 by Max Lewis. He focused on the production of clothing for sale to tourists and some of the earliest proto-Hawaiian shirts (with labels), come from Royal Hawaiian Manufacturing. This company was bought out by Watumull's in 1955.[38]

Women's Attire

Unique silhouettes, transformed from a wide variety of ethnic influences invigorated women's designs in the 1930s. Most of women's wear was made at home or in custom dress shops (such as Margo's), although the amount of clothing imported from America increased.

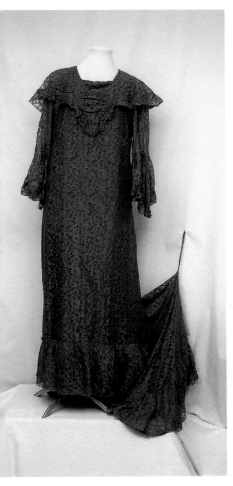

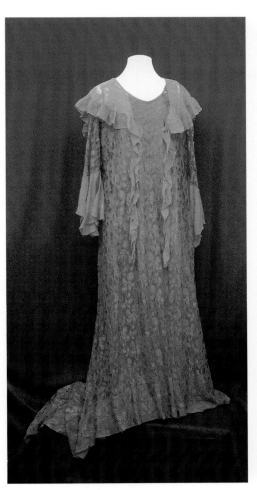

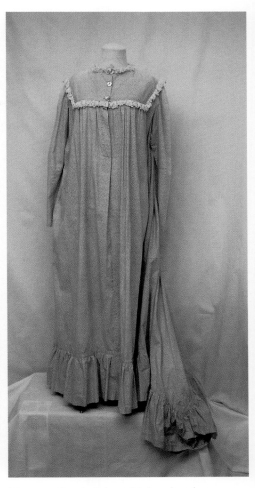

Lace and silk holoku, 1930s, 98.2.5, $700 to $999

Lace over silk holoku, 1930s, 98.2.6, $700 to $999

Cotton calico holoku with handmade lace, 1930s, 83.5.3, $700 to $999

Hawaiian designs were influenced by Asian and Western design elements. Like the palaka shirt before it, the lauhala hat moved from functional work clothing to high fashion. This was due to the influence of Elsie Krassas, one of the first fashion designers in Hawai`i. She began her career in 1933 by designing lauhala hats (papale) to be worn by women. Originally, lauhala hats were worn by men and women for functional purposes; these had high crowns and flat or rolled rims. Krassas designed hats to be worn with fashionable women's dress, and trimmed them with kapa, wooden roses, shells and other items from the local environment.

While the traditional loose style of holoku continued to reflect consistency and tradition, the fitted holoku, was highly influenced by western fashion and became a favorite style of younger women. Bias cuts and zippers were added for a snug fit. In 1937, Elsie Krassas turned to the holoku and streamlined the garment. She modeled it at garden parties and holoku balls. This modernized holoku was rapidly adopted by the fashionable set.[39]

The mu`umu`u was still considered to be an undergarment or housedress and worn only at home. It was generally made in light colored cottons, in either solids or small prints. The garment was also worn by local folks for swimming, rather than swimsuits. It was not until the invention of Hawaiian prints, and the use of them in constructing mu`umu`u in the 1940s that the dress was considered acceptable for public wear.

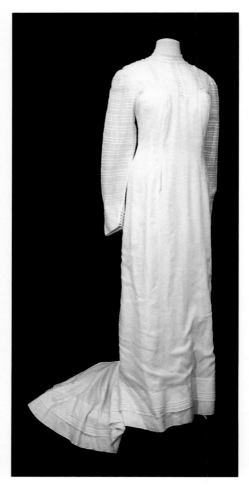

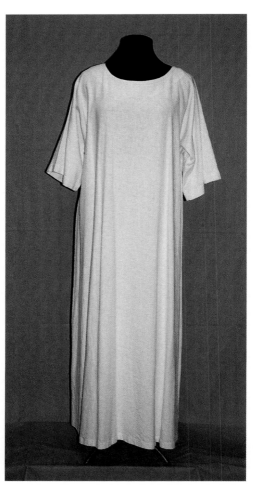

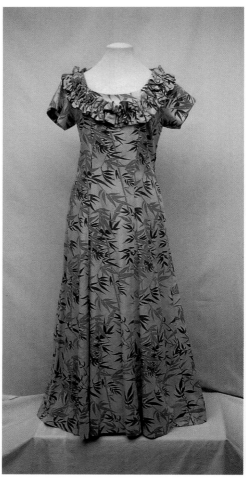

White cotton lawn holoku, 1930s, 93.1.2, $700 to $999

Cotton homespun fabric, reproduction of 1930s mu`umu`u, 89.11.1, under $100

Cotton broadcloth mu`umu`u, late 1930s, 76.28.1, $700 to $999

Men's Wear: The Aloha Shirt

Contrary to what is in print in other books on the Hawaiian shirt, the aloha shirt was *not* developed in the 1920s or even in the 1930s. While the predecessors of the Hawaiian shirt were established by the mid 1930s, what is recognized around the world as the early Hawaiian shirts – the brightly patterned rayons with Hawaiian motifs— are shirts that were created *after* World War II. As explained in more detail earlier, the dominant fabric found in shirts of the early 1930s was a plain cotton broadcloth, usually with a white background and only one or occasionally two other colors in the print. They were made in a pullover style with three button tab front closures and were worn by both men and women. "In the 1930s we wore white shirts in town until they invented Aloha Week." Hawaiian motifs did not appear on the early aloha shirts until 1935, and when found, these were extremely simple designs. It was not until the late 1930s that tropical motifs were attempted for aloha shirts; these were the shirts made of drapery fabric.[40]

George Brangier, and his partner Nat Norfleet, started their company Branfleet (later Kahala Sportswear) in 1936 and sold these kimono-cloth predecessors to aloha shirts that were being sold by others as well.[41] These shirts were reported to have been made by Japanese mothers out of silk and crepe kimono fabric scraps for their school children. Similarly, reports exist that boys from an upper-class private school began having shirts made of bright kimono fabric to wear for special activities, but the most common explanation has been that families had matching shirts made of bright kimono fabrics for special events.

In the mid-1930s the word 'aloha' was attached to many types of merchandise- there were 'aloha' tea sets and 'aloha' coasters, so the term was not only used for sportswear. The first to use the term in ads was Musa-Shiya the Shirtmaker who advertised in 1935 in the Honolulu Advertiser on June 28, 1935, "Aloha shirts — well tailored, beautiful designs and radiant colors." However, it was Ellery Chun who trademarked the term 'aloha shirt' in 1936. He too began by selling shirts made of traditional kimono fabrics although he wanted to produce an expressly Hawaiian shirt. He commissioned artists (notably his sister, Ethyl Lum) to create Hawaiian designs of local flowers and fish, and had these designs printed on kabe crepe. Because they sold well, Chun noted that: "I figured it was a good idea to own the trademark."[42]

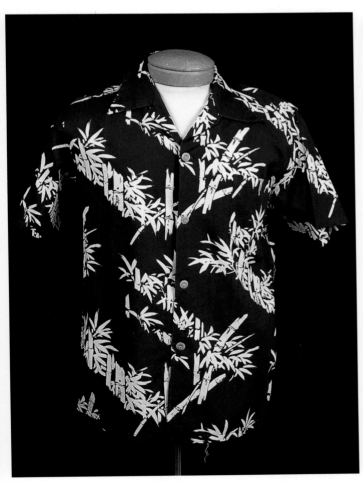

Early 1930s aloha shirt of yukata fabric from Japan with bamboo buttons, 95.2.11, $1,000+

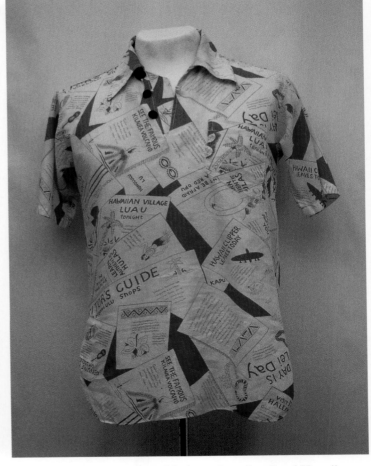

1937 aloha shirt, cotton broadcloth tourist print, *Royal Hawaiian Manufacturing Co.*, 98.14.6, $1,000+

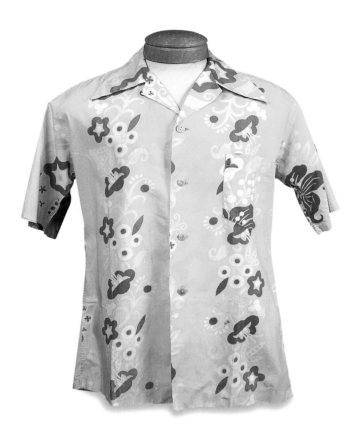

Cotton border print, plastic buttons, 1938, 76.27.8, $1,000+

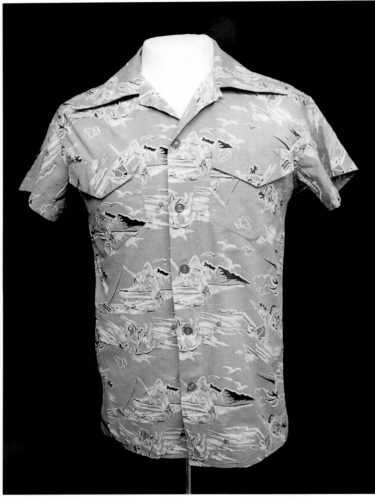

Early 1940s aloha shirt, cotton print of keiki (children) fishing, pocket flaps, plastic buttons, 99.1.2, $700 to $999

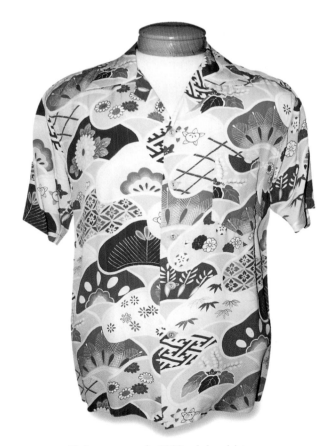

Kabe crepe early 1930s aloha shirt, bamboo buttons, 95.2.1, $1,000+

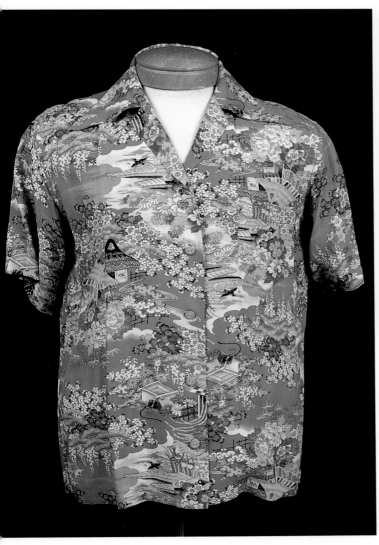

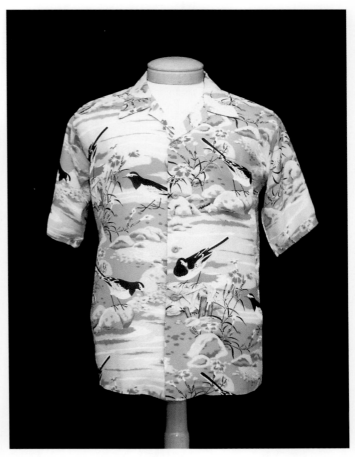

Kabe crepe from Japan. Early 1940s, 95.2.4, $700 to $999

Kabe crepe early 1930s aloha shirt, bamboo buttons, 95.2.6, $1,000+

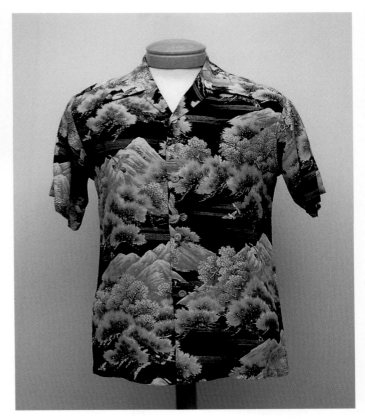

Kabe crepe from Japan, 1940s, 95.2.3, $700 to $999

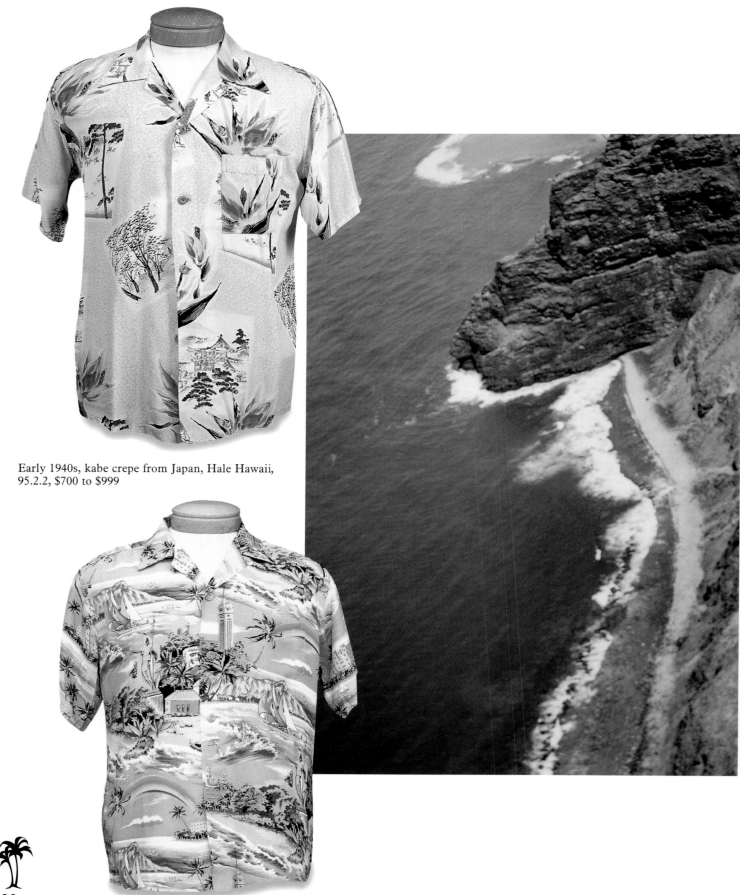

Early 1940s, kabe crepe from Japan, Hale Hawaii, 95.2.2, $700 to $999

Early 1940s, kabe crepe from Japan, *Reef*, 85.16.2, $1,000+

5. The Post-War 1940s To Mid-1950s
Classic Silkies

Cultural Context

After textile imports ceased during World War II, the creation of uniquely Hawaiian textiles began out of necessity in Hawai`i. Artists began designing textiles with tropical motifs for garments. In the early 1940s aloha shirts were made from drapery remnants. These are among the earliest tropical print aloha shirts. The drapery shirts produced by Wong's Draperies were a local phenomenon; they were only worn by local residents, never by tourists. Although these drapery shirts were not advertised, they remained popular from the 1940s through the 1960s and even became popular in America as Hawaiian students went to college on the mainland, then sent home a request for Wong's shirts. They were heavy cotton and comfortable for football games.[43] Nonetheless, drapery shirts were a bit warm for Hawai`i. The tropical designs were in great demand so the design motifs were scaled down, and the designs were printed on softer, more comfortable material — rayon. Historical motifs were added to the designs as well. Consequently the bright, bold rayon aloha shirts, known to collectors around the world as Hawaiian shirts, originated in the post-War 1940s. The brightly patterned rayon aloha shirt became famous throughout the nation as servicemen returned home from Hawai`i, and tourism increased through the mid-twentieth century. The 1940s and 1950s were the heyday of Hawaiian tourism. Hawaiian fabrics were used extensively in Hawaiian apparel both for sale to tourists and to the Hawaiian-born population.

In 1946 the Honolulu Chamber of Commerce appropriated $1,000 to study aloha shirts and prepare suitable designs for clothing businessmen could wear during the hot summer months. A resolution was passed that allowed the City and County of Honolulu employees to wear sport shirts from June through October each year, but the aloha shirt was excluded. The resolution allowed for "open-collar sport shirts in plain shades, but not the ones with the loud colorful designs and patterns." In 1947 the first Aloha Week was established. City employees were then allowed to don aloha shirts for business, but only during the single week each year.

Aloha Week arose from an uneasy mixture of cultural and economic motives. A Honolulu businessman named Harry Nordmark felt that Hawaiian cultural practices needed to be re-instituted. 'I thought it was a pity that none of this pageantry was left,' Nordmark recalled, ' the glory of ancient Hawai`i was behind museum walls. The public was forgetting that such music, dancing and philosophy of life ever existed.'[44] The first Aloha Week brought pageantry back to the people; it was in October 1947 at Ala Moana Park which was close to Waikiki.

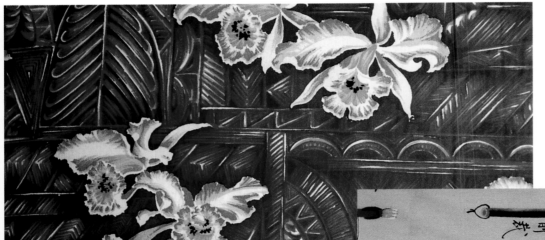

Cotton, *Shaheen's* Orchid Tapa.

Cotton fabric by *Malihini*, Calligraphy tools motif.

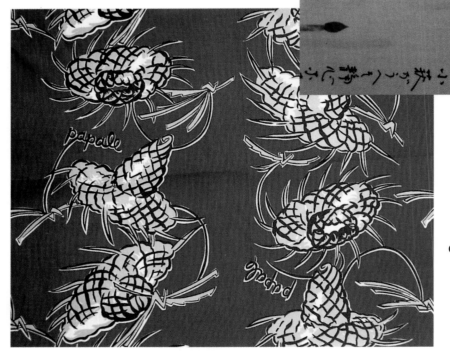

Cotton fabric of papale (lauhala hats).

Volunteers built an authentic Hawaiian village. There were ancient Hawaiian sports, a holoku ball, a floral parade, and a makahiki festival. More than 8,000 people showed up for the makahiki festival, which featured hundreds of Hawaiians playing the parts of royalty in the pageant. Economically, the development of Aloha Week was a sound business decision. It was scheduled for October, a slow month for tourism, and it was designed to attract visitors. Another beneficiary was the Hawaiian fashion industry, which produced mu`umu`u and aloha shirts to be worn during Aloha Week. This festival now lasts from September through early November, with events scheduled on all islands. The institution of Aloha Week in 1947 led to the demise of drab businesswear through a permanent adoption of aloha shirts as business dress.[45]

Fabrics

Due to the scarcity of imported fabrics and clothing, aloha attire became more popular on the Islands for the local population during the War. For some time, tourists and military personnel had readily adopted aloha shirts, but due to a lack of other options, the local Islanders began to accept them as well. Locally produced fabrics in Hawaiian prints were sewn into women's wear as well. The mu`umu`u was no longer seen as a housedress once it was made of Hawaiian prints. Similarly, holoku were produced in Hawaiian prints during the War and post-War years.

The dominant fabrics used for women's wear between 1945 and 1958 were made of cotton or silk. The high-end manufacturers used combed cottons, which have a fine texture. Rayon fabric became commonly used after World War II. Rayon, a regenerated cellulose, was named in 1924 and took three decades to develop into a usable fabric.[46] Rayon came into wide use in the late 1940s, and was primarily used for aloha shirts. Several of the manufacturers in the pre-War period avoided using rayon because, as one noted "The rayon was garbage ... It was flimsy and inexpensive. ... they came out with a rayon that was heavier, and it finally held the dyes. Rayon shirts with a smooth finish and Hawaiian prints were only seen after World War II. No one was printing that stuff before the War."[47]

The heavy rayon fabrics described above felt like silk, hence the nickname, "silkies", a term adopted in the 1960s. These shirts were designed with bold colors and brilliant tropical designs, often done in "hash" prints - where assorted motifs were randomly thrown onto a fabric. Mu`umu`u, sarong dresses and aloha shirts made of rayon during this time period are highly collectible. During the mid 1940s, Hawaiian designers began creating textiles for clothing since they could no longer import fabric. "During the war when Japanese imports were no longer available, Hawaiian prints came into their own" according to Kamehameha's owner, Herb Briner.[48]

Hawaiian textile art, especially the most outrageously designed, has been appreciated by connoisseurs for several decades. A few artists produced huge designs in which the entire shirt was treated like a canvas. Some of these featured air-brushed designs of Polynesian maidens. Tourism created a ready market for more adventurous aloha attire by the post-World War II era. Designs grew more daring, incorporating such uniquely Pacific patterns as palm trees, hula girls, Diamond

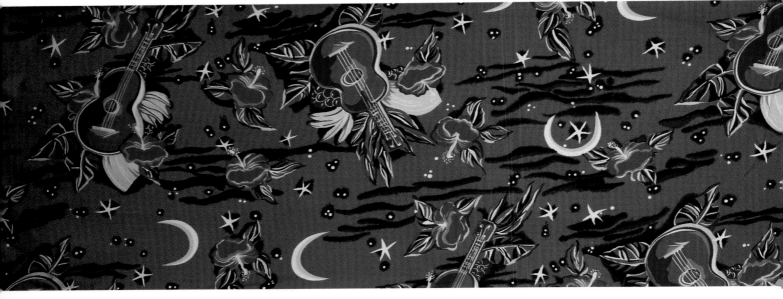

Rayon, late 1940s.

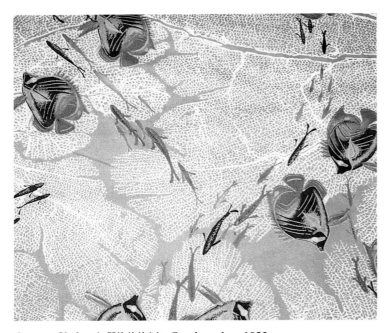

Cotton, *Shaheen's* Kihikihi in Coral garden, 1952.

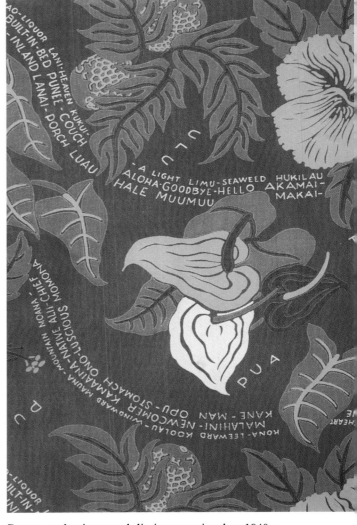

Rayon, anthuriums and dictionary print, late 1940s.

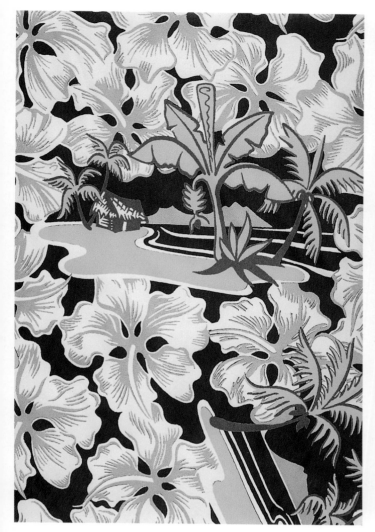

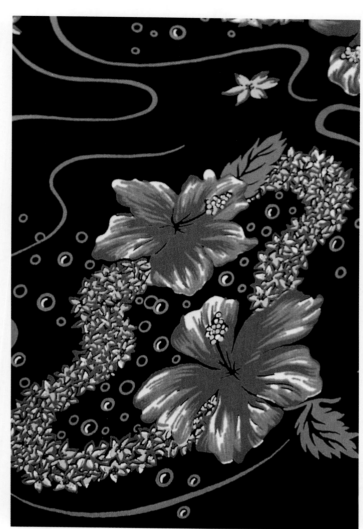

Rayon, late 1940s

Rayon, late 1940s.

Head, the Aloha Tower, surfers, and pineapples. Color combinations
were no longer staid; colors became riotous. School children waged
contests to see who could find the most outrageous outfit, and soon
entire families were wearing the shirts, often in matching prints. Fabric became art because professional artists were brought in to create
the Hawaiian designs. Alfred Shaheen was the first manufacturer to
professionalize the textile arts:

> I got together a group of artists ... They'd been living hand
> to mouth, barely surviving. And I put them in a studio and put
> them on salary and taught them to do textile design – it's an
> art all in itself because the design had to be done in repeats and
> color separations had to be done for each one. I usually had
> four textile designers. ... What I did was to make my designs
> more demonstrative. I'd have my artists go into the Bishop
> Museum and study the kapa, and look for artifacts that could
> be illustrated. Basically what I wanted them to do was to create
> a textile design that had some meaning to it, not just doodling
> on fabric like everyone else was doing, throwing on a surfboard
> and palm tree and so forth. So we tried to put more substance
> into the design, and on the hangtag we'd write the story be-
> hind the design.[49]

John Meigs was a painter who was fascinated by kapa designs. He
began designing artwork for the major producers, and also did designs

37

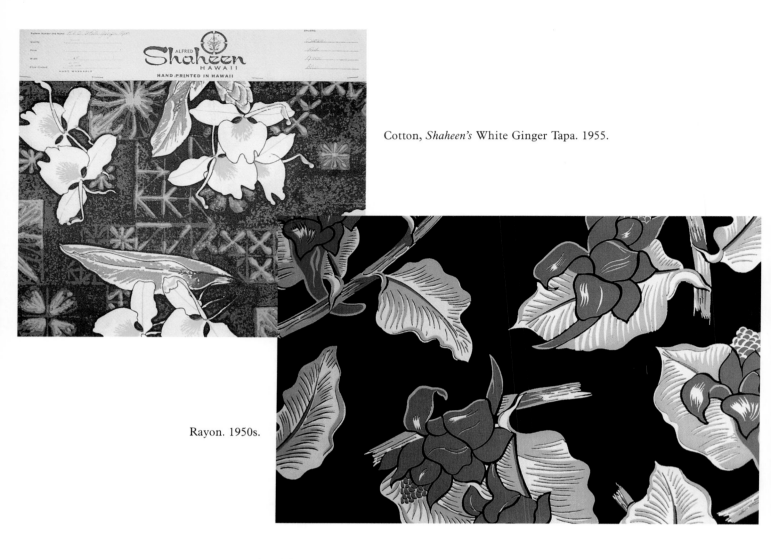

Cotton, *Shaheen's* White Ginger Tapa. 1955.

Rayon. 1950s.

under his Hawaiian name, Keoni. While there are no surviving examples of his designs based on kapa, which he created in 1939, aloha shirts with his designs utilizing motifs relating to other aspects of Hawaiian culture, flora and marine life are in private collections. Keoni's later work (from the late 1940s through 1951) foreshadowed the beginnings of abstract art in Hawaiian textile design.

Handprinted fabrics produced under the Surf 'n Sand Label were done by Shaheen's crew of designers between 1947 and 1955. Some of these were on rayon. By the late 1950s, rayon was no longer being used in aloha attire. This was obvious from the number of well-documented aloha shirts in the University of Hawaii's Ethnic Costume Collection, but was clarified by Alfred Shaheen, a manufacturer of the time period, who stated: "The idea that they quit using rayon due to a fire at duPont is a myth. Rayon became old hat – it simply went out of style. Period." The gaudy floral designs were considered too garish and were no longer fashionable. Funderburke notes "Cotton has been the primary fabric used for prints of Hawaiian fabric designs."[50] In the late 1950s blended fabrics of cotton and arnel came into being and the promise of permanent press fabrics brought cottons with synthetic blends into style.

Clothing Production

In the late 1940s and early 1950s, major retail stores on the mainland promoted Hawaiian-made garments. Filene's of Boston claimed to have had "the largest exhibit of Hawaiian material ever assembled outside the Islands." This kind of attention, coupled with the introduction of air traffic between Hawai`i and the US mainland resulted in the air transport of garments from Kamehameha and Kahala to Boston via Pan American World Airways and American Airlines. Several garment companies began business and aimed at both the local Hawaiian market as well as the mainland US market. In 1946, Malihini Sportswear was incorporated to manufacture apparel for both men and women. This family run business is still in operation, and designer Ray Sasaki consistently produced aloha attire that is not of the run-of-the-mill tourist stereotype.[51] By aiming at a more global vision of sportswear, as did Shaheen and later Tori Richard, these companies remained successful.

Aloha Week had an impact on clothing in Hawai`i, in that aloha attire became more in demand by local consumers. While at first that demand was for clothing for local people to wear to the festivals, over time people began to wear aloha attire more frequently. Local manufacturers found this to be a positive move, in that they had begun to fear that conventional mainland modes of dress might supplant island garb.[52]

Alfred Shaheen worked for a few years in the custom dress business with his parents and formally started in 1947 with the registration of his label Surf n' Sand. He set up his aloha shirt business in 1948 with four machines and six employees, and soon expanded to producing women's wear as well as aloha shirts. Most of the fabric was printed in the US and brought to Hawai`i through the Panama Canal. Manufacturers had to keep large inventories on hand. "By the time the Korean situation hit in 1950, I'd been doing aloha shirts for two years. I had about a four month supply of fabric" at which time the value of that inventory dropped by more than half. "I barely survived financially. I said to myself — this is ridiculous — if I am gonna stay in this business I have got to control the fabric." And he did just that, by developing unique textile printing techniques. Shaheen was noted for his fashion-forward women's wear designs. He became the largest apparel manufacturer in the next two decades because of his ability to produce unique and innovative textile designs primarily done on combed cottons.[53]

Iolani started to manufacture clothing in 1953. Although the firm was primarily noted for the manufacture of men's shirts, by 1959 they had about 30 percent of their production in women's wear. Many of the company designs featured hand-screened panels as decorative accents and their clothing was targeted toward the local population rather than tourists. Their shirt designs were subdued, often in plain colors, with simple designs often on the pocket.

Women's Attire

Aloha attire, as a term, originated in the 1950s, with mu`umu`u, holomu`u and aloha shirts seen as a unique category of apparel. Women in the Islands tended to wear mu`umu`u at home for casual wear, and, in public, tended to favor conservative, western-styled clothing rather than Hawaiian prints until the 1950s. "They were very conservative and still had the missionary influence. The formal aspect of dress was a remaining influence of the missionaries" said Alfred Shaheen, who

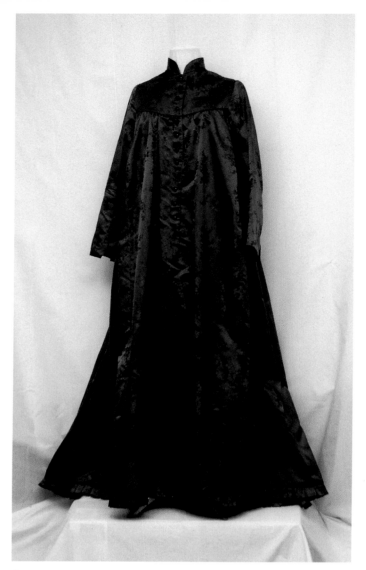

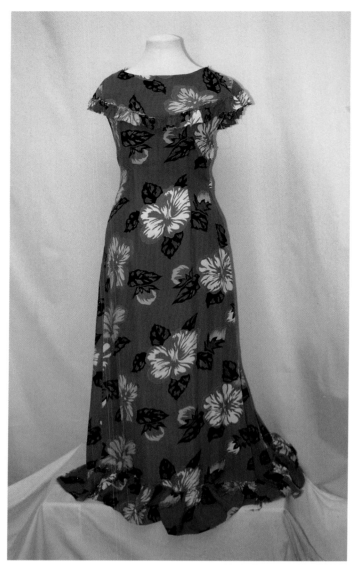

Custom made holoku of Chinese silk in 1945, *Toshimi of Waikiki*, 87.11.1, $700 to $999

Late 1940s custom made rayon holomu`u, 79.24.2, $700 to $999

single-handedly made the holomu`u famous. The holomu`u was invented in 1949 as a combination of the holoku and mu`umu`u; it could easily be worn during the day because it lacked a train, but it had the close fit that young women were looking for. To that, beautiful Hawaiian prints (such as Shaheen's pareau print) were added and the holomu`u was well positioned to be the darling of the entertainment industry.

However, conservatism in Island dress was about to be changed by designers such as Bob Sato, who designed for Alfred Shaheen, and Elsie Krassas. Her tropical prints for interior design were such a hit that in 1940 she scaled down the designs and created bright Hawaiian textiles for women's beach wear and play clothes; designing for movie stars made her famous.[54] Once Hawaiian prints were available for apparel, they became commonly found on both holoku and mu`umu`u; by putting bright prints on the mu`umu`u it was freed from the confines of the home and considered appropriate to wear in public. The mu`umu`u was loose and casual, and worn long. During the post-War period, there was a great deal of entertaining on the islands, and the favored garment for parties (as well for entertaining in the tourist industry) was the holoku which had become more fitted. Trains lengthened to enormous proportions. Reverence for the holoku as an elegant garment, reflecting the elegance of a bygone era in Hawaiian history, continued unabated through the 1940s and into the 1950s.

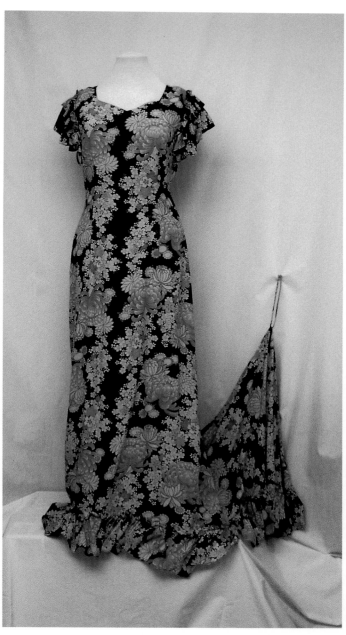

Japanese kabe crepe holoku, *McCully Square* Dressmaker, late 1940s, 76.39.4, $700 to $999

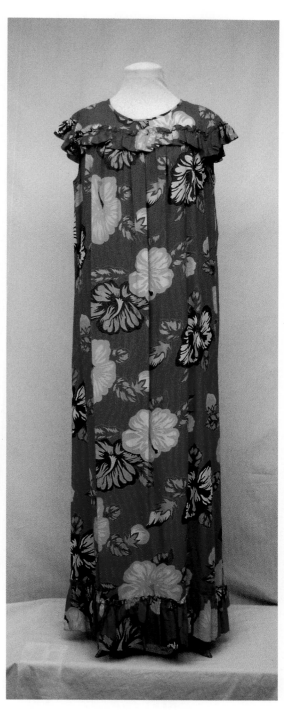

Rayon mu`umu`u, custom made, 1940s, 76.39.3, $700 to $999

41

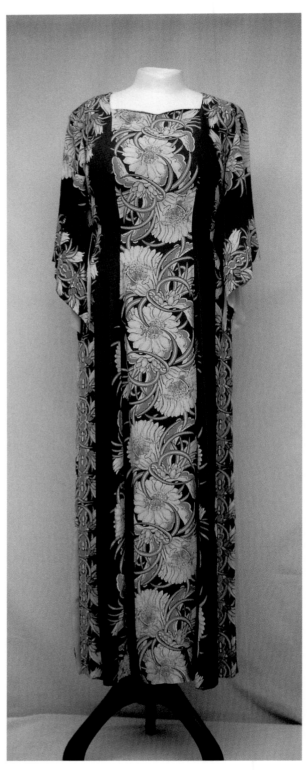

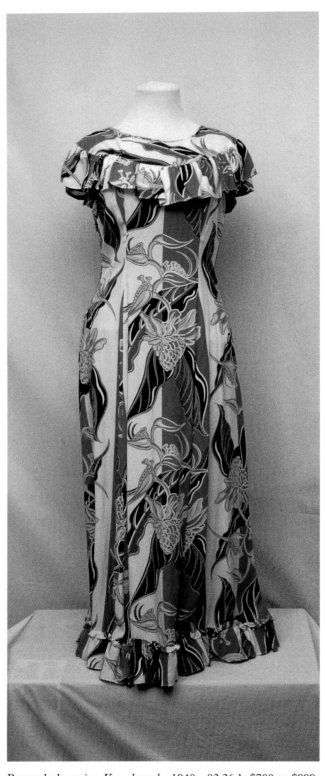

Rayon pake mu`u, made with *Shaheen* fabric, 1940s, 88.3.1, $700 to $999

Rayon holomu`u, *Kamehameha,*1940s, 82.26.1, $700 to $999

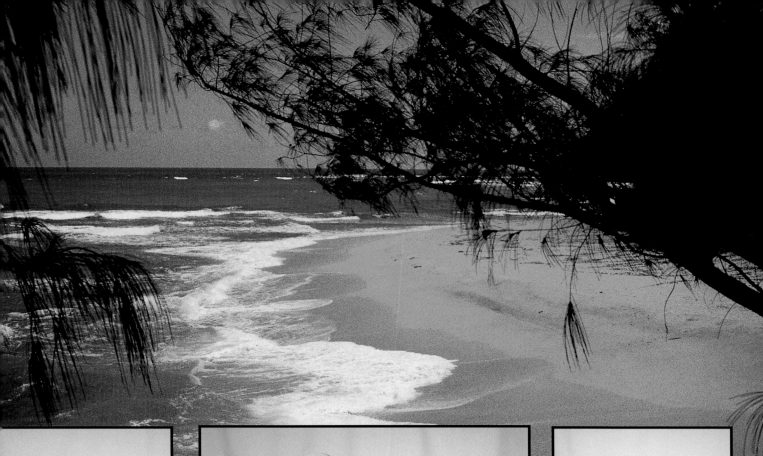

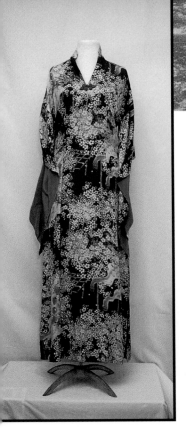

Silk pake mu`u, *Kuhio Sportswear*, 1940s, 98.2.10, $700 to $999

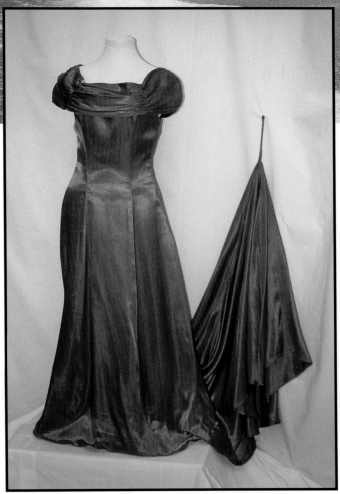

Silk satin holoku, worn by 1948 queen of the Aloha Festival, 82.6.1, $700 to $999

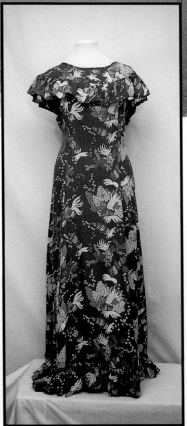

Rayon holomu`u, *HoAloha*, 1950s, 98.2.12, $300 to $699

43

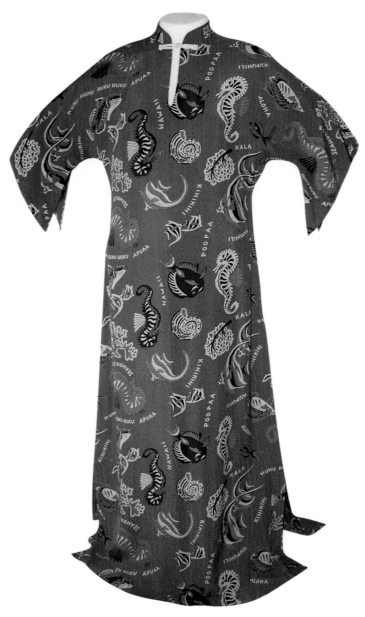

Rayon pake mu`u, *Shaheen*, 1950s, $700 to $999

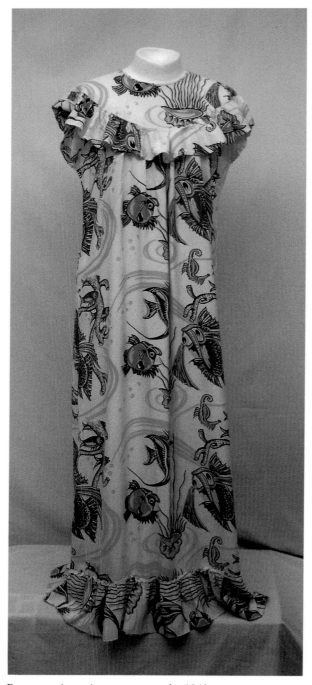

Rayon mu`umu`u, custom made, 1940s, 85.5.4, $700 to $999

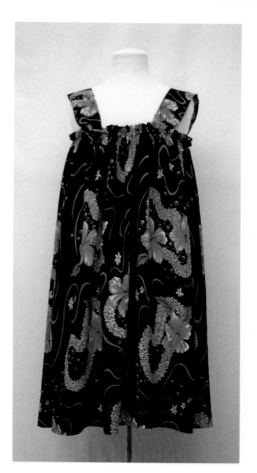

Rayon mu`umu`u, custom made, 1940s, 76.29.8, $300 to $699

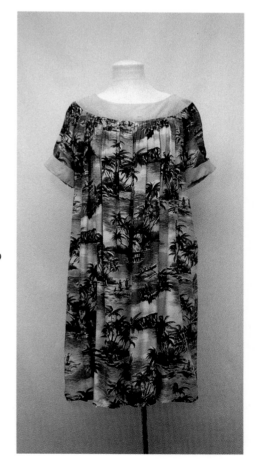

Custom made rayon mu`umu`u, 1940s, 98.14.2, $100 to $299

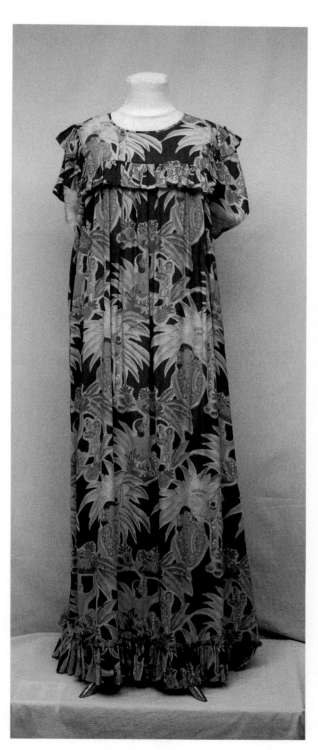

Rayon mu`umu`u in Matson menu print by Frank MacIntosh, Custom made, 1950s, 76.39.2, $700 to $999

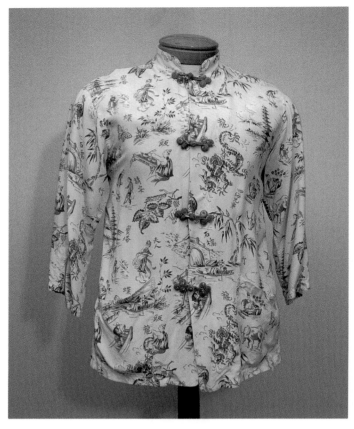

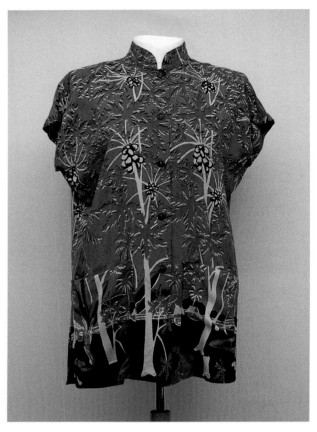

Rayon woman's pake aloha shirt, Chinese frog closures with pockets at hem, 1940s, 81.13.2, $700 to $999

Rayon woman's pake aloha shirt, *Royal Hawaiian Manufacturing Co.*, 1940s, 98.14.3, $700 to $999

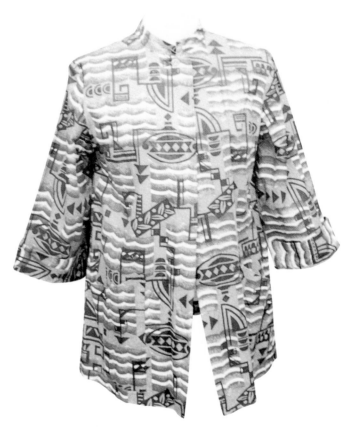

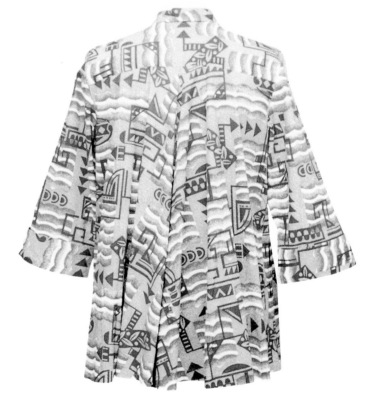

Cotton aloha shirt jacket. Front view. *Royal Hawaiian Manufacturing Co.*,1940s, 99.2.1, $300 to $699

Cotton women's aloha shirt -swing jacket style. Back. *Royal Hawaiian Manufacturing Co.*, 1940s, 99.2.1, $300 to $699

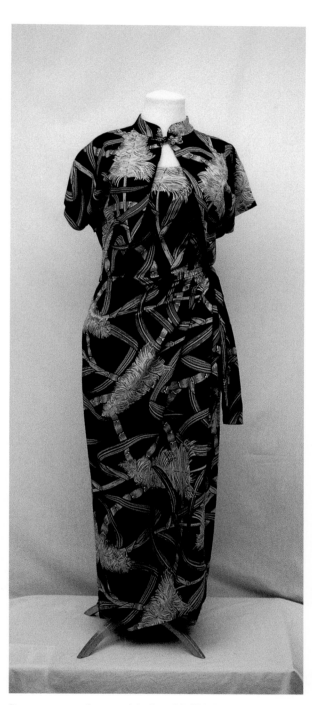

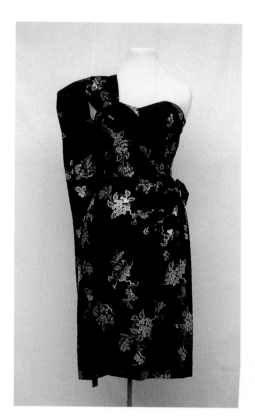

Sarong dress, manufactured by *Elsie Krassas* of fabric designed in 1954 by *Shaheen*, 79.18.1, $100 to $299

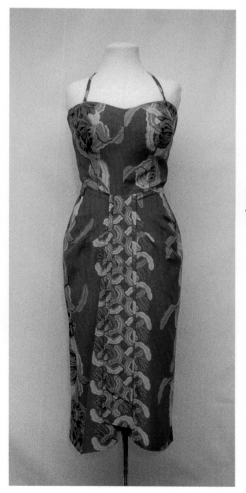

Rayon sarong dress, *Shaheens of Honolulu*, 1950s, 89.3.1, $100 to $299

Rayon sarong dress and jacket, *Malihini*, 1948-50, 73.1.3, $300 to $699

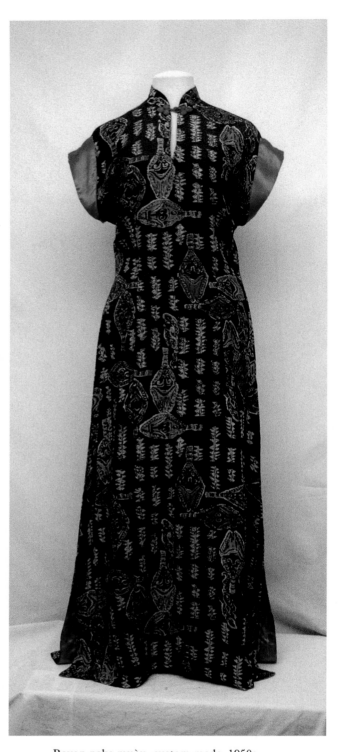

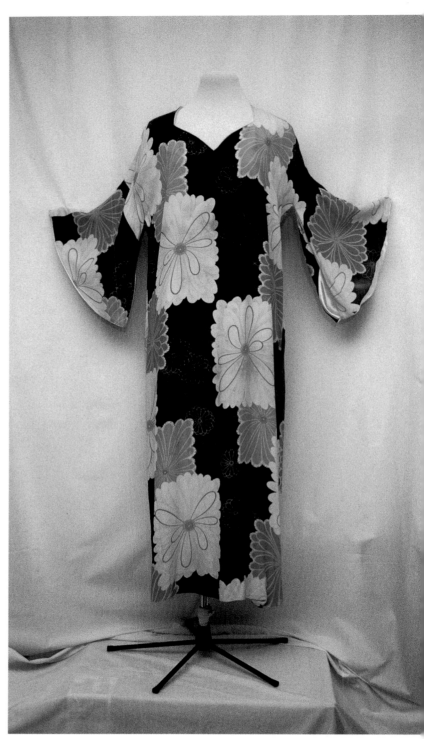

Rayon pake mu`u, custom made, 1950s, 89.7.1, $700 to $999

Rayon pake mu`u, *Hata Dry Goods, Hilo*, 1950s, 76.26.2, $700 to $999

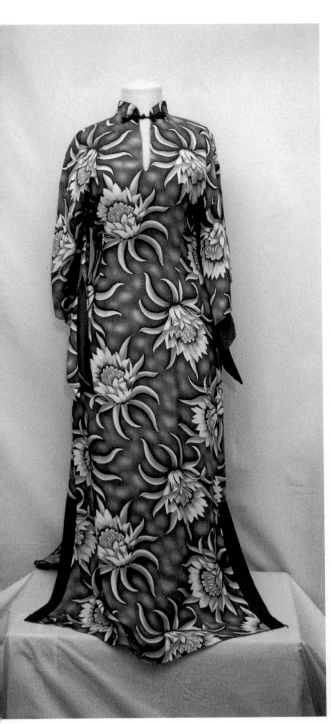

Rayon pake mu\`u, *Royal Hawaiian Manufacturing Co.*, 1950s,
80.3.1, $300 to $699

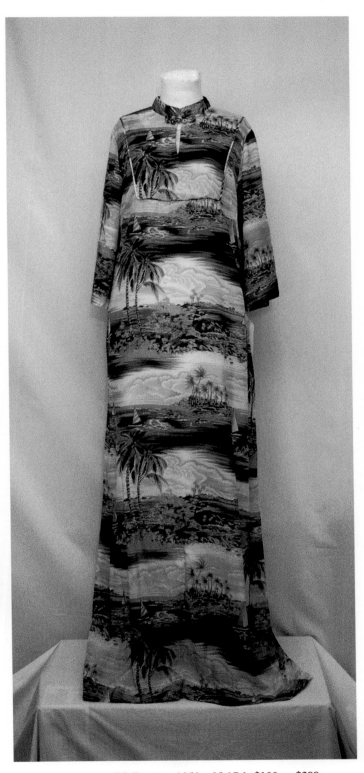

Rayon pake mu\`u, *JC Penneys*, 1950s, 85.17.1, $100 to $299

49

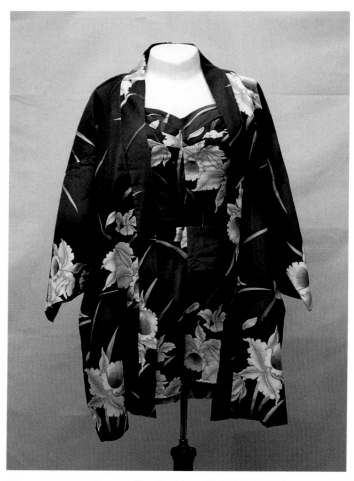

Cotton sateen swim set, *Sun Fashions (Kahala)*, 1953-56 98.13.5, $100 to $299

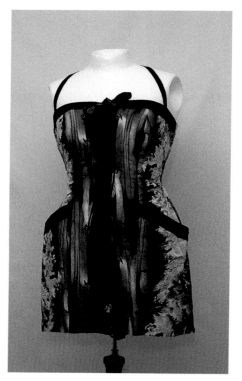

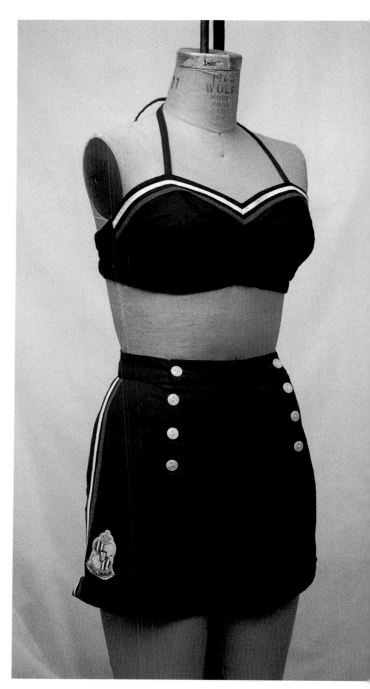

Sailor Moku swimsuit, cotton, *Royal Hawaiian Manufacturing Co.*, 1940s, 95.6.36, $300 to $699

Cotton swimsuit, *Kamehameha, Made in Hawaii*, 1950s, 94.5.1, $100 to $299

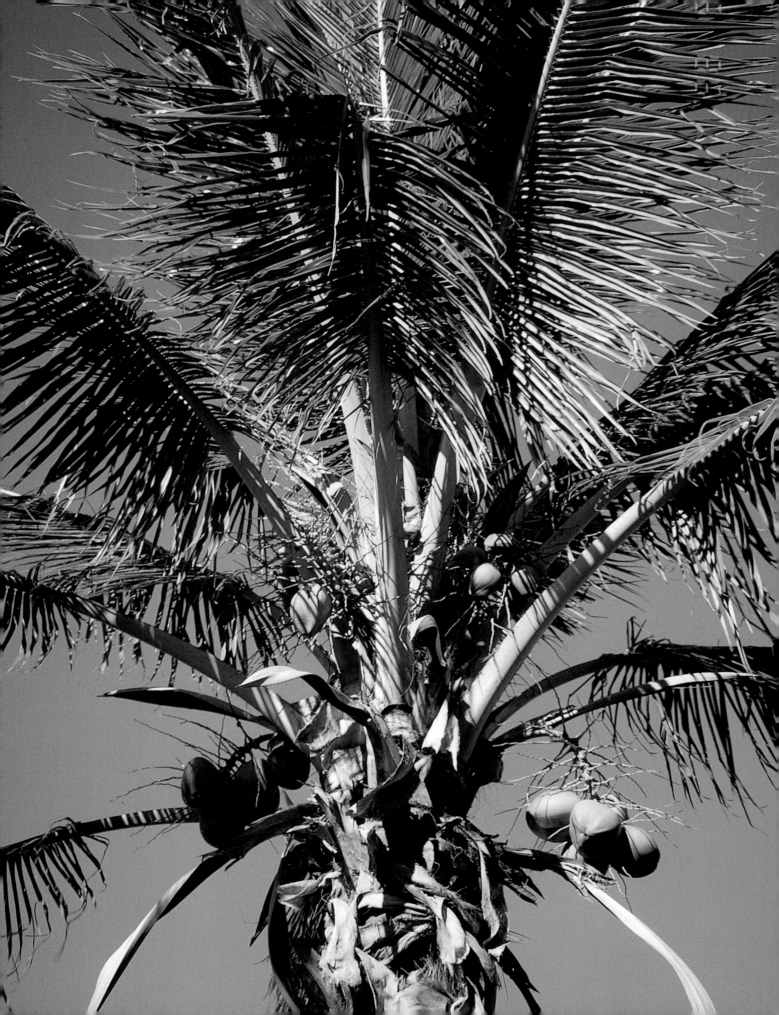

Men's Wear

The aloha shirt became the ultimate picture postcard representing exotic, tropical vacations on the Islands. Out-of-towners continued to comprise a large part of the buying public until World War II when exports were halted. Locals bought the shirts to support the economy, and members of the armed forces who were stationed in Hawai`i snatched up dozens of the colorful keepsakes during their tenure in the tropics. President Harry Truman, and entertainer Arthur Godfrey made public appearances in aloha shirts, stimulating their popularity. Apparel manufacturers had generally bought their fabric from the US mainland, but these textile companies required runs of at least 10,000 yards. Japanese mills had minimum runs of just 3,000 yards, so until the War, Hawaiian manufacturers often obtained yardage from Japan. The cessation of imports and exports during World War II created drastic changes in the aloha shirt industry. A major manufacturer of aloha shirts noted:

> During the War there was one or two million servicemen in Hawai`i who were introduced to the Islands. Some stayed and married, others went home and then came back with wives. They introduced the aloha shirt to the mainland. ... This was about 1950 when tourism started to be important. We weren't a tourist market yet because there were only three or four hotels then. There was a craze for Hawai`i on the mainland then, related to the push for statehood in the US Congress.[55]

The aloha shirt became a hot commodity and travelers often took aloha shirts home with them. Textile design included Hawaiian language, historical sites, flowers and cultural motifs. Kamehameha Garment Company accomplished an impressive feat in 1951 by producing the seven-color reproduction of the Eugene Savage Matson menu painting for prints on sportswear. "We (Kamehameha, Shaheen, Branfleet) had been shipping shirts to the mainland but then the mainland shirt makers got into it. Cisco manufactured shirts with Duke Kahanamoku's name and with the movie "From Here to Eternity" aloha shirts exploded on the fashion scene."[56]

Montgomery Clift, Frank Sinatra and Ernest Borgnine were dressed in aloha shirts from the 1950s, even though the movie was supposed to be set in 1941. According to a garment manufacturer of the time, the movie's costumer bought the shirts in Honolulu, right off the rack in 1954.[57] Numerous mainland publications in 1950 featured Duke Kahanamoku's introduction of aloha shirts produced by Cisco. In a 1950 publicity photo with Arthur Godfrey, Duke wore a shirt that would later become famous in the 1954 film "From Here to Eternity." This shirt has been incorrectly dated in other books due to confusion over the licensing of Duke's name. Duke Kahanamoku licensed his name three times; it was not until the second time - 1950 - that Duke's name was connected to the shirt later worn by Montgomery Clift. Publicity photos of the release of Duke Kahanamoku shirts on the mainland, printed in the New York Post and the Daily Compass clearly date this shirt to January, 1950.[58]

> "The new Duke Kahanamoku line of aloha shirts and beach shorts for men, manufactured by the Cisco Company of New York, was presented to the New York Press yesterday [1/21/50] at the Stork Club... The print patterns are all Hawaiian in

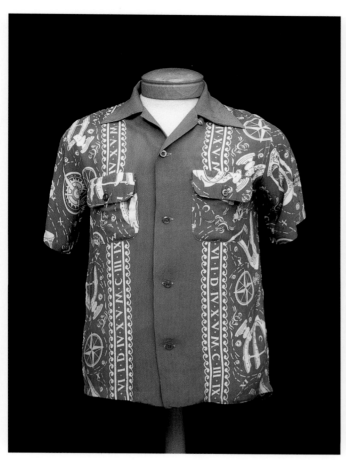

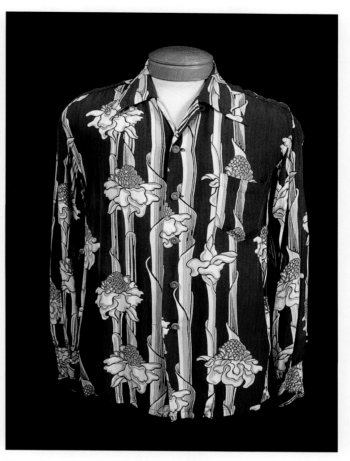

Rayon aloha shirt, custom made, 1940s, 97.11.7, $700 to $999

Rayon long-sleeved aloha shirt, torch ginger pattern, *Kamehameha*, late 1940s, 87.8.2, $1,000+

origin, and suggest a good approach to Hawaiian flavor via fabric, for women's as well as men's fashions. These aloha shirts look as though they could also be merchandised as beach shirts for women to coordinate with the [aloha] shirts. The grounds are usually dark brown, red or navy and the pattern is white, sometimes introducing a third color."[59]

Aloha shirts were still seen as casual dress, not appropriate for the business world until after World War II. Aloha Week brought about change. Until then, men in Hawai`i wore shirts with ties to work. There was a lot of resistance to wearing aloha shirts for anything but casual wear. "It was really provincial in Hawai`i then, the old timers were into formality. They weren't far from the missionaries, in fact many were descendants of the missionaries so they were still pretty strict and puritanical about things" said a manufacturer. "These were the top guys in business – haoles - who ran things. So it was a new breed, the younger guys who were ready for a new shirt style."[60] Well into the late 1950s the City and County of Honolulu insisted this stylish sportswear was not acceptable dress for its 5,000 male employees, even during the sticky summer months. In 1954, some local businesses began to encourage broader use of the aloha shirt. Employees were asked to wear aloha shirts throughout the humid summer, but cautioned that they be "clean and tucked-in." The editor of the newspaper expressed hope that other businessmen would join in wearing local attire.[61]

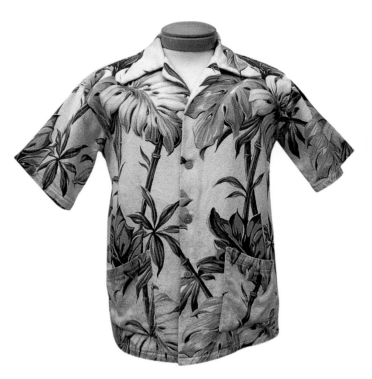

Cotton barkcloth (drapery fabric) aloha shirt, *Wong's Drapery,* 1948, 98.14.1, $700 to $999

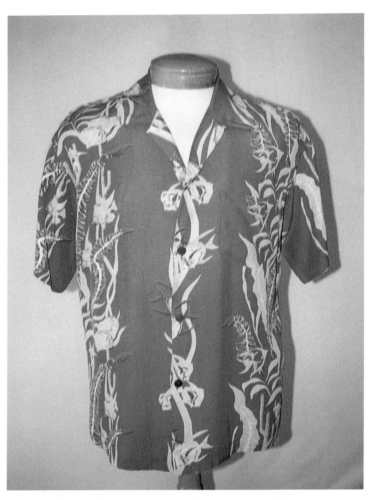

Rayon aloha shirt, late 1940s, *Andrade,* $1,000+

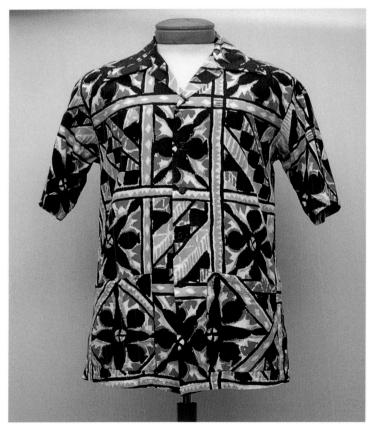

Cotton aloha shirt, *Shaheen's,* 1948-1949, 76.27.7, $700 to $999

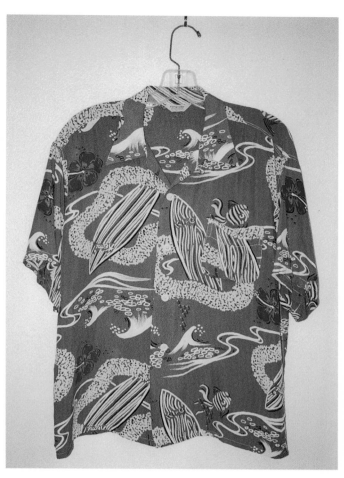

Rayon aloha shirt, *Keoni of Hawaii*, by *Kuonakakai*, 1951,
$700 to $999

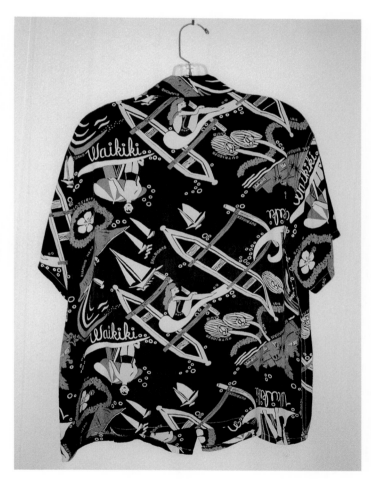

Rayon aloha shirt, *Keoni of Hawaii*, Manufactured by *Pilgrim*,
1951, $1,000+

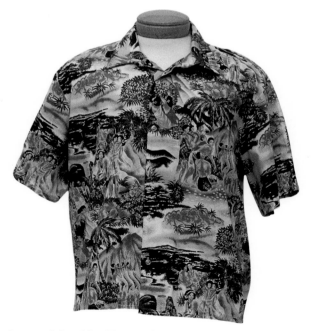

Cotton aloha shirt, Eugene Savage print, *Kamehameha*,
Courtesy of Kamehameha Garment Co., $300 to $699

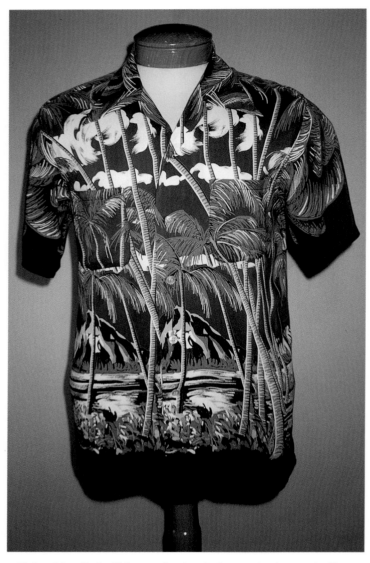

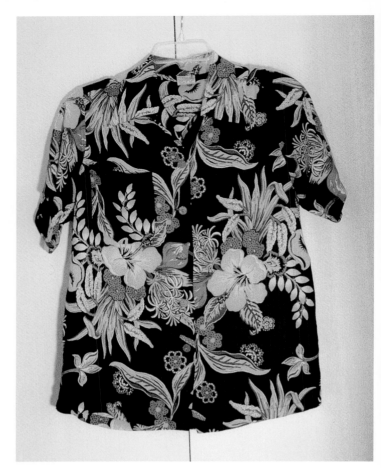

Rayon aloha shirt, *Surf n' Sand (Shaheen), Courtesy of Camille Shaheen-Tunberg,* 1953, $1,000+

Aloha shirt, *Duke Kahanamoku,* (made famous in the movie *From Here to Eternity*) 1951-1955, $1,000+

Cotton aloha shirt, kapa design, *Shaheen's of Honolulu, Courtesy of Camille Shaheen-Tunberg,* 1952-1957, $300 to $699

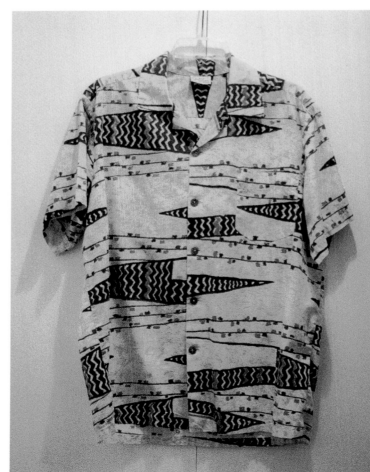

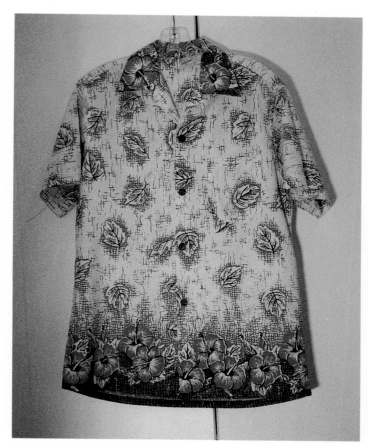

Cotton aloha shirt, hibiscus design, *Shaheen's of Honolulu, Courtesy of Camille Shaheen-Tunberg,* 1953, $300 to $699

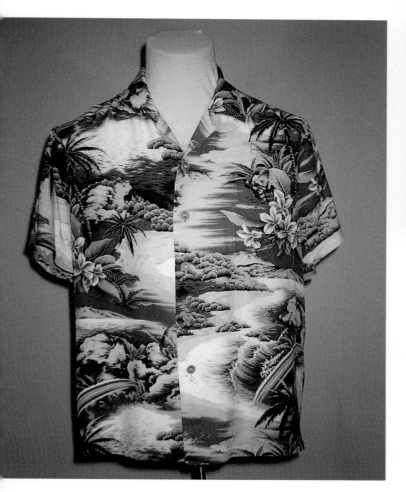

Rayon aloha shirt, palm tree design, *Malihini,* 1950s, 73.1.8, $700 to $999

Rayon aloha shirt, rainbow design, *Pali Style Hawaiian,* 1950s, $700 to $999

Rayon aloha shirt, lei design,
Watumull's, 1950s, $1,000+

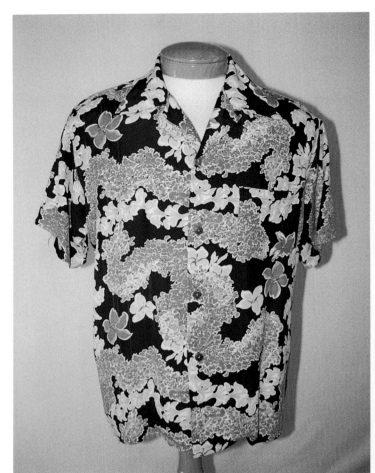

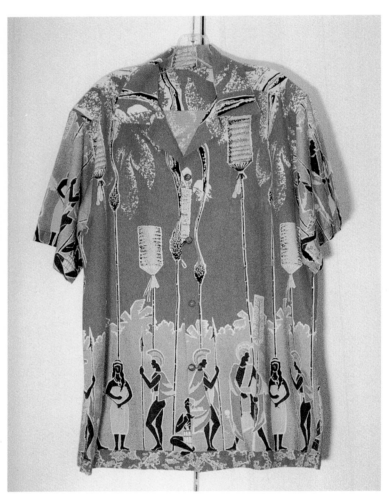

Cotton aloha shirt, ali'i with kahili design, *Shaheen's of Honolulu,*
Courtesy of Camille Shaheen-Tunberg, 1954, $1,000+

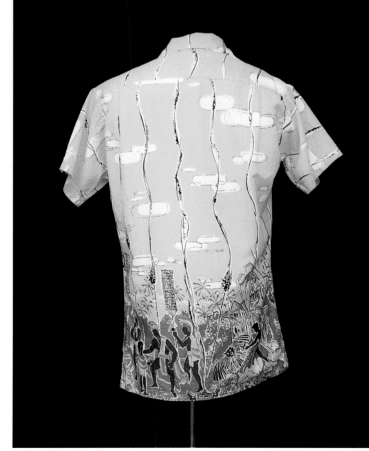

Cotton aloha shirt, *Shaheen*
yardage,1955, 87.12.9, $700 to $999

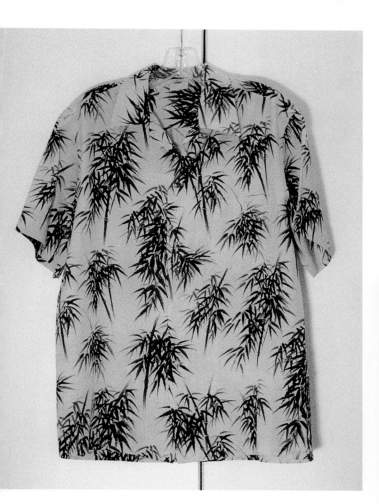

Silk pongee aloha shirt, *Shaheen's of Honolulu, Courtesy of Camille Shaheen-Tunberg*, 1954, $300 to $699

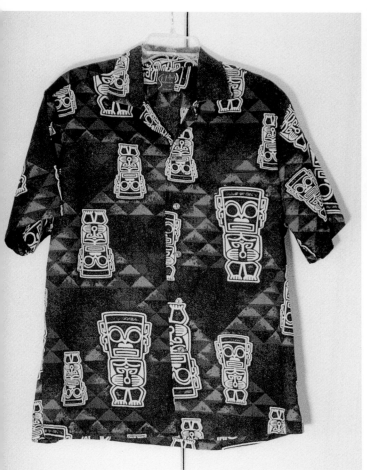

Silk aloha shirt, *Poi Pounder*, 1950s, 97.11.5, $1,000+

CST7, 1955, aloha shirt, blue/white, cotton, *Shaheen's of Honolulu*, Courtesy of Camille Shaheen-Tunberg, $300 to $699

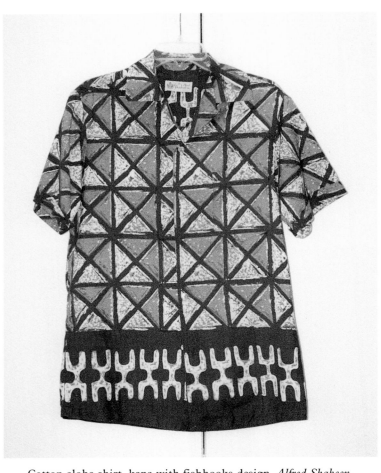

Cotton aloha shirt, kapa with fishhooks design, *Alfred Shaheen, Courtesy of Camille Shaheen-Tunberg*, 1955, $300 to $699

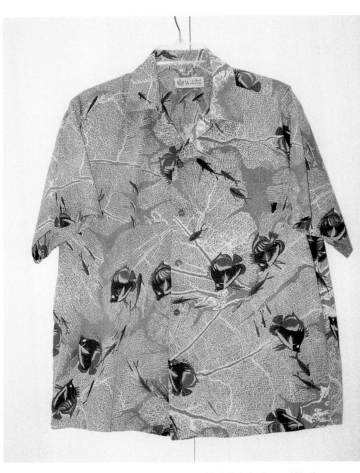

Cotton aloha shirt, coral fantasy with kihikihi design, *Alfred Shaheen, Courtesy of Camille Shaheen-Tunberg*, 1955, $300 to $699

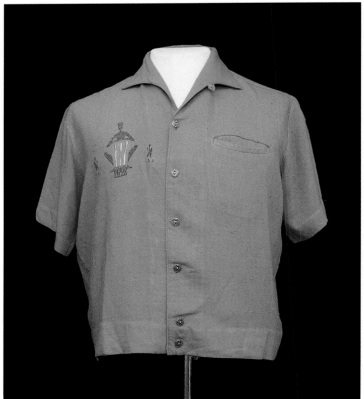

Cotton aloha shirt, *Hawaiian Surf- Pacific Sportswear*, 1950s, 76.27.11, $700 *to* $999

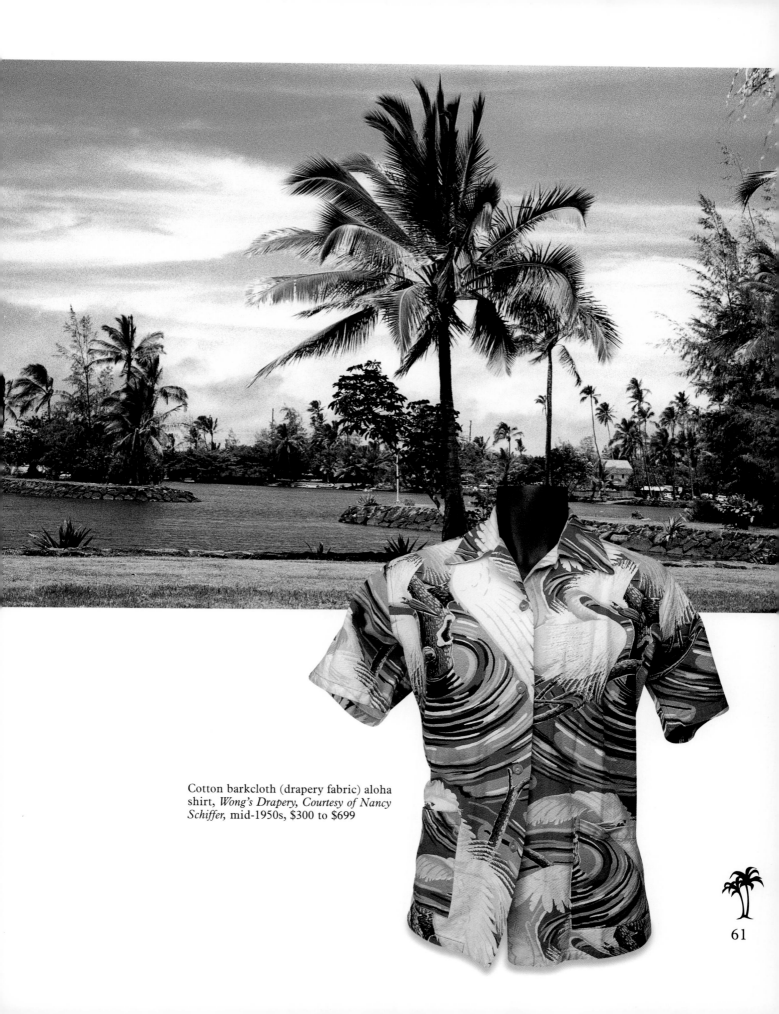

Cotton barkcloth (drapery fabric) aloha shirt, *Wong's Drapery, Courtesy of Nancy Schiffer,* mid-1950s, $300 to $699

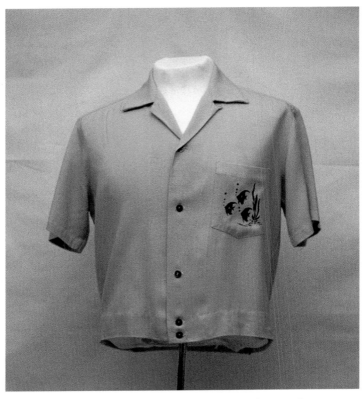

Cotton aloha shirt, *Iolani*, 1950s, 98.14.4, $700 to $999

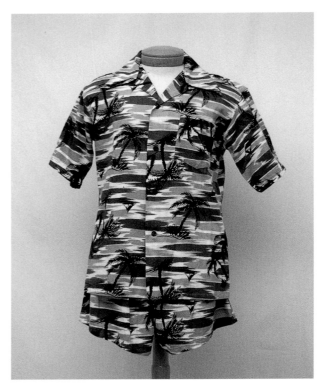

Cotton cabana set, *Malihini*, mid-1950s, 76.27.5, $700 to $999

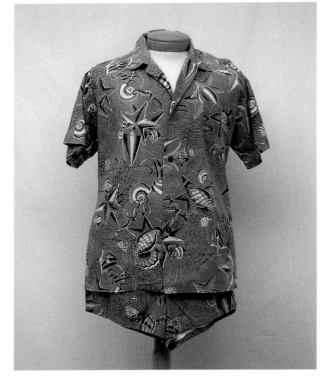

Cotton cabana set, *Shaheen's of Honolulu*, mid-1950s, 94.2.1 , $300 to $699

6. The Late 1950s
An Era Of High Fashion

Cultural Context

The 1950s reflected a constant push toward westernization in Hawai`i; after half a century as an American territory, Hawai`i ended the decade by becoming a state in 1959. During this time, the garment manufacturing industry nearly tripled sales due to the increased national interest in Hawai`i, as statehood was discussed in Washington DC. Sales promotions by national and local manufacturers pushed casual wear in conjunction with the growth of suburban living, and the growing tourist trade was just about to take off. "Most of the fashion business at that time was the carriage trade. You had the winter tourists who stayed at the Royal Hawaiian but tourism wasn't a year round industry yet and there were only a few hotels."[62] Hawai`i still had the allure of a vacation destination for the rich. When the Surfrider Hotel opened in 1951, followed by the opening of the Princess Kaiulani, Biltmore and Hawaiian Village Hotels in 1955, tourism increased substantially.[63]

The exoticism of Hawai`i captured the nation's imagination. Movies had a huge impact with at least one blockbuster per year set in the Islands. Hawai`i became a state on August 21, 1959 after several years of promotion in the US Congress. As a result of the constant media attention, the years just before and after 1959 represented a time when Hawai`i had the nation's attention. A mu`umu`u fad in colleges on the mainland kept the focus of garment production on Hawaiian-Polynesian styles. "Aloha attire became important in the 1950s" said Alfred Shaheen, "it was when mu`umu`u, holomu`u and aloha shirts became a whole way of dressing." Competition, especially from California, became a problem and Hawaiian manufacturers began to insert "Made in Hawai`i" labels into their aloha wear. This was a successful campaign, and sales of aloha attire increased once again. The most successful manufacturers, notably Shaheen and Tori Richard, did not rely on aloha attire for their company's bottom line; they took a more global approach by designing and producing garments for the mainland and Europe as well.

Fabrics

Shaheen created the most innovative textiles in Hawai`i during this time period and had a huge impact on both the garment industries in Hawai`i and on the mainland. He created textiles for his company, but also produced for other manufacturers as well as producing yardage for the home sewer.

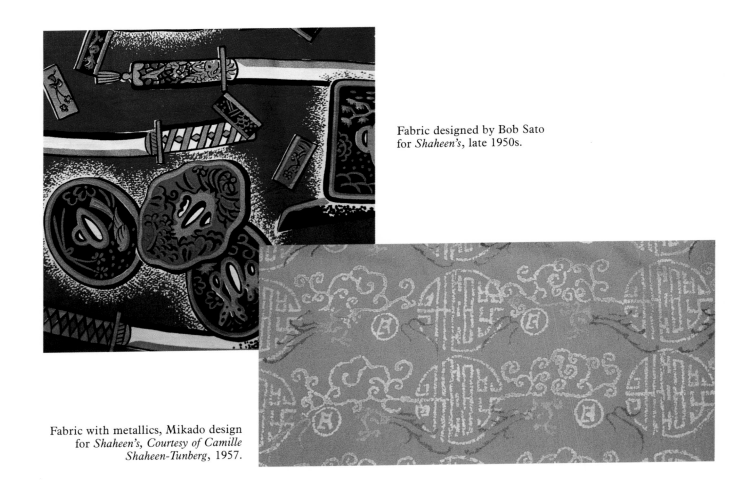

Fabric designed by Bob Sato
for *Shaheen's*, late 1950s.

Fabric with metallics, Mikado design
for *Shaheen's, Courtesy of Camille
Shaheen-Tunberg*, 1957.

I bought the goods plain, white, and prepared for printing.
I ordered 100,000 yards at a time because it was woven to my
specifications. So what I had in inventory was plain goods. I
didn't print until I needed it; I never got stuck with inventory
— that is what happens when you buy 10,000 yards or even
3,000 yards. I had sixteen 60-yard silk-screening tables that
turned over four times a day – close to 4,000 yards in an eight-
hour shift.

Bob Sato, the lead textile designer was "like my hands," said
Shaheen as he explained how Sato would produce designs that Shaheen
had in his mind. "We would work together, Bob and I, and usually
four other textile designers, and Richard Goodwin, who designed the
garments. We worked in mylar, and metallics to produce garments for
Surf n' Sand," the Shaheen label for Hawaiian garments. Shaheen's
designs were copied by many other designers and fabric makers. He
produced exclusive fabrics for specific retail outlets, such as Liberty
House, McInerny's and Sears (which was then considered upscale).

In the late 1950s, a resurgence in interest in kapa was seen in textile design. Textile artists studied artifacts and incorporated this imag-
ery into textile design. Alfred Shaheen took his designers to Asia, Tahiti and other locations to study the material culture of Polynesian
islands and Asian cultures. From this exposure, they created designs
with Asian and Polynesian elements and stimulated a trend for
Polynesian and Asian-inspired textiles. In 1958, Shaheen began to create engineered prints to make it harder for his designs to be copied by
Japanese textile firms. Engineered prints are designed so that the pattern is not interrupted by the garment's style lines. The earliest engineered prints in Hawai`i were borders and panels.

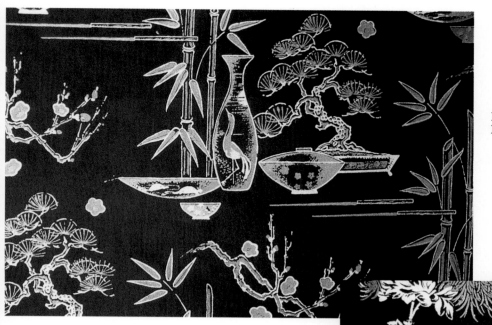

Fabric with metallics, designed by
Bob Sato for *Shaheen's*, late 1950s.

Chrysanthemum design on cotton by
Bob Sato for *Shaheen's*, late 1950s.

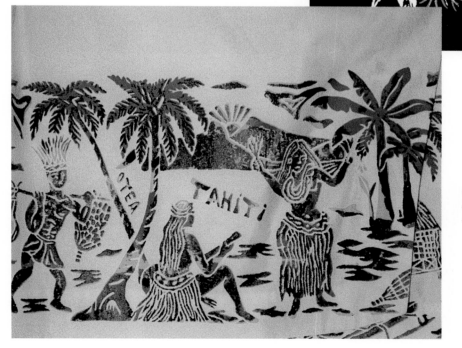

Cotton blend Tahiti design for
*Shaheen's, Courtesy of Camille
Shaheen-Tunberg*, late 1950s.

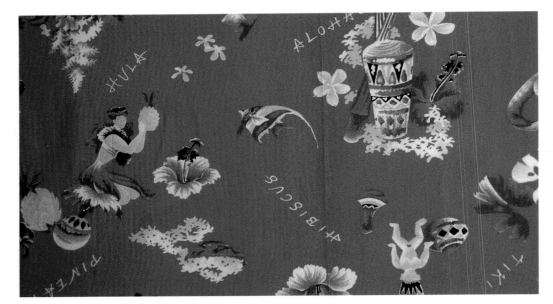

Cotton blend fabric, Lei and Tiki design, 1959.

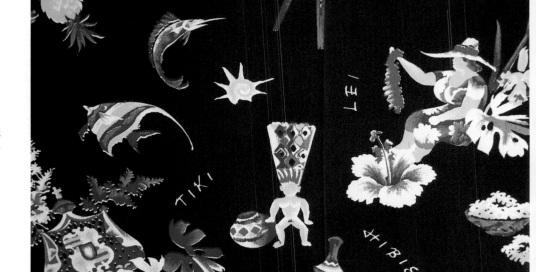

Cotton blend, Lei and Tiki design, 1959.

Clothing Production

The late 1950s through the 1960s was a period of unprecedented growth for the Hawaiian fashion industry. Just before the War, sales were at roughly $50,000 year. By 1947 volume was up to $2.5 million. Referring to the mid-1950s, Shaheen stated that

There was no industry in Hawai`i then, and I was the only one hiring and I was hiring lots of people. So the mayor and the governor were all real interested in what I was doing because there was real potential for growth. ... So I brought models to Hawai`i and had a fashion show in the factory, to show the bankers, builders and other guys what was possible. I was revolutionizing the business – I brought in section work, modeling, and unique textiles and garments.

Following the War, sales of apparel increased approximately 30% annually until 1961. Sophisticated resort wear, manufactured by companies like Shaheen and Tori Richard, drove the industry to be the third largest exporter in Hawai`i. Mort Feldman and his wife Janice

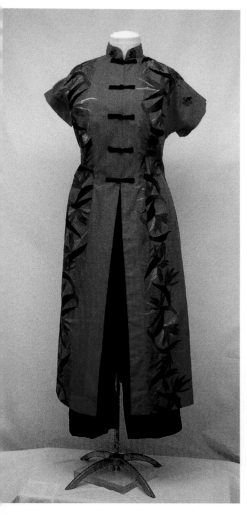

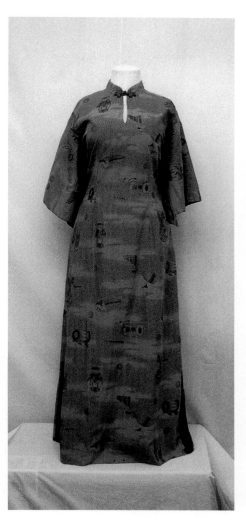

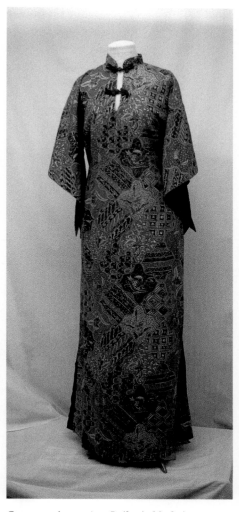

Cotton tea timer, Custom made, 1955, 76.39.5, $300 to $699

Cotton pake mu`u, *Hawaiian Casuals by Stan Hicks*, late 1950s, 88.4.1, $300 to $699

Cotton pake mu`u, *Leilani, Made in Hawaii*, , 1956, 94.2.7, $100 to $299

named the company (Tori Richard) after two of their children. Established in 1956, Tori Richard produced most of its garments for women until they began making shirts in 1973. When he came to Hawai`i from Chicago, Feldman wanted to create a look that was sophisticated; like Shaheen they both parlayed their mainland garment industry experience into a resort-wear niche that paid off in the long run. While both companies produced aloha attire, it was just a portion of their overall production, which allowed them to survive the cyclical nature of aloha attire fads.

Women's Attire

By the late 1950s, aloha attire had become just as commonly seen in Honolulu as garments imported from the States. Leisurewear was a new category; popular styles were tea timers (Chinese-influenced pant and jacket set); Hawaiian swimsuits, mandarin-style sheath dresses (modeled after the cheong sam) with Suzie Wong side slits.[64] The loose, brightly patterned and often short mu`umu`u became associated with

casual day wear, and the pake mu`u was a closer fitting mu`umu`u
with a mandarin collar. Pake jackets, with Chinese knot buttons down
the front and two patch pockets were also popular for casual wear. For
evening, cocktail dresses made in Hawaiian fabrics but with mainland
styles (such as halter-top dresses) along with and the holoku, dominated for formal evening wear. The fitted holoku became the favored
style for special events in Hawai`i. Hawaiian prints and extremely long
trains were popular on the holoku of the 1950s. Long sleeves and yokes,
which had formerly characterized the traditional holoku, became less
common. Modesty became less of a concern, as women's shoulders
and chests were bared for the first time since the missionary's cam-
paign to completely cover Hawaiian women's bodies in the nineteenth
century. Backs were also exposed in the 1950s. The holomu`u became
very popular in the 1950s. Designed as a more casual garment than the
holoku, the holomu`u retained the close fit of the holoku but elimi-
nated the train. "Holoku had two different types of trains; a peacock

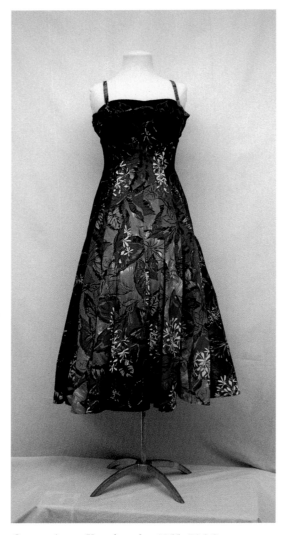

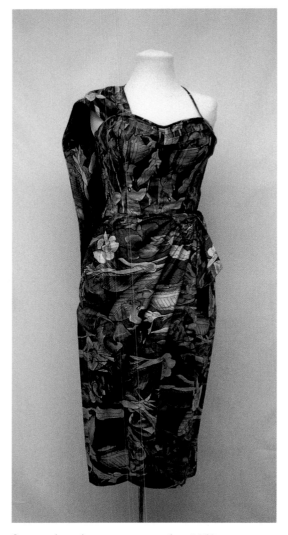

Cotton dress, *Kamehameha*, 1955, 74.8.2,
$100 to $299

Sarong dress in cotton sateen, late 1950s,
98.8.93, $100 to $299

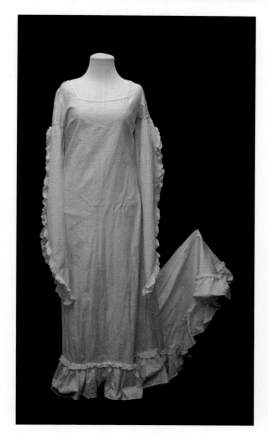

Cotton sateen custom made holoku, late 1950s, 97.9.3, $100 to $299

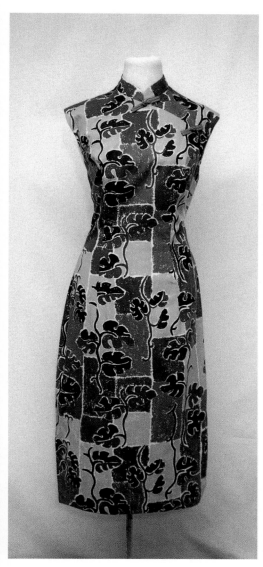

Susie Wong mu`umu`u in cotton, *Kamehameha,* late 1950s, 86.8.51, $100 to $299

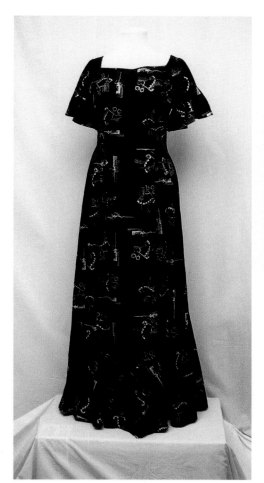

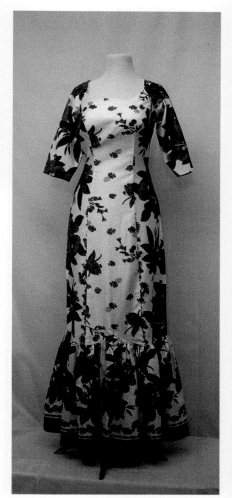

Cotton sateen holomu`u, *Kamehameha* 1958, 98.15.1, $100 to $299

Cotton holomu`u, *HoAloha,* late1950s, 78.6.1, $300 to $699

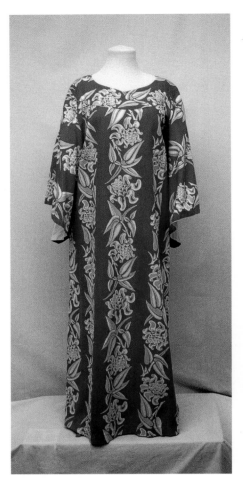

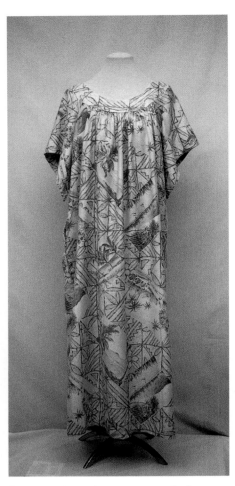

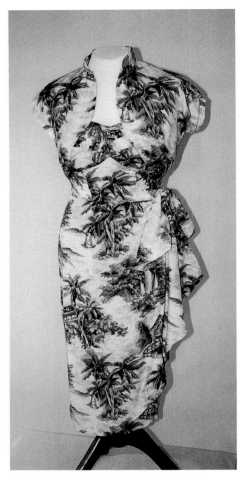

Cotton muʻumuʻu, custom made, 1955, 89.4.3, $700 to $999

Cotton muʻumuʻu, custom made, late 1950s, 97.15.2, $100 to $299

Rayon sarong dress, *Lauhala*, 1950s, $700 to $999

train or fishtail train. Mother [owner of Margo's, a custom dress business] used to make holoku of slipper satin or lace and so forth and I made the holoku and holomuʻu; I was known for the holomuʻu because the entertainers liked the way I could get it to skim the body."[65]

In 1958, Bete Incorporated was founded by Betty Manchester who had worked for McInerny's, Leilani Shops, and Kahala Sportswear, Ltd. Betty continued her interest in clothing construction with training at the University of Hawaiʻi. When she decided to create her own line of women's apparel, she chose the Hawaiian spelling of her name, "Bete," thinking it more appropriate for a collection of muʻumuʻu. Before creating her designs, Betty did research both at the Bishop Museum and in family scrapbooks. A 1905 photograph of a Hawaiian woman in a high-necked, long dress had the caption in her father's writing, "Hawaiian woman selling strings of flowers." These turn of the century holoku captured her imagination. In the late 1950s, the Bete muʻumuʻu was a radical change from popular bright Polynesian prints that changed every year. Instead, Bete designed four muʻumuʻu and made them of calico prints so the resulting garments resembled the 1905 photo. Sold under the Bete label to the better department and women's stores, Bete's garments have been associated with kamaʻaina and have a missionary flavor. In 1961, Bete made a black velvet muʻumuʻu for Jackie Kennedy Onassis soon after John Kennedy's inauguration. Many Island women bought muʻumuʻu in the same style but in a calico print. The original designs are still being produced; these garments fit exceptionally well, and are still popular in Hawaiʻi today.

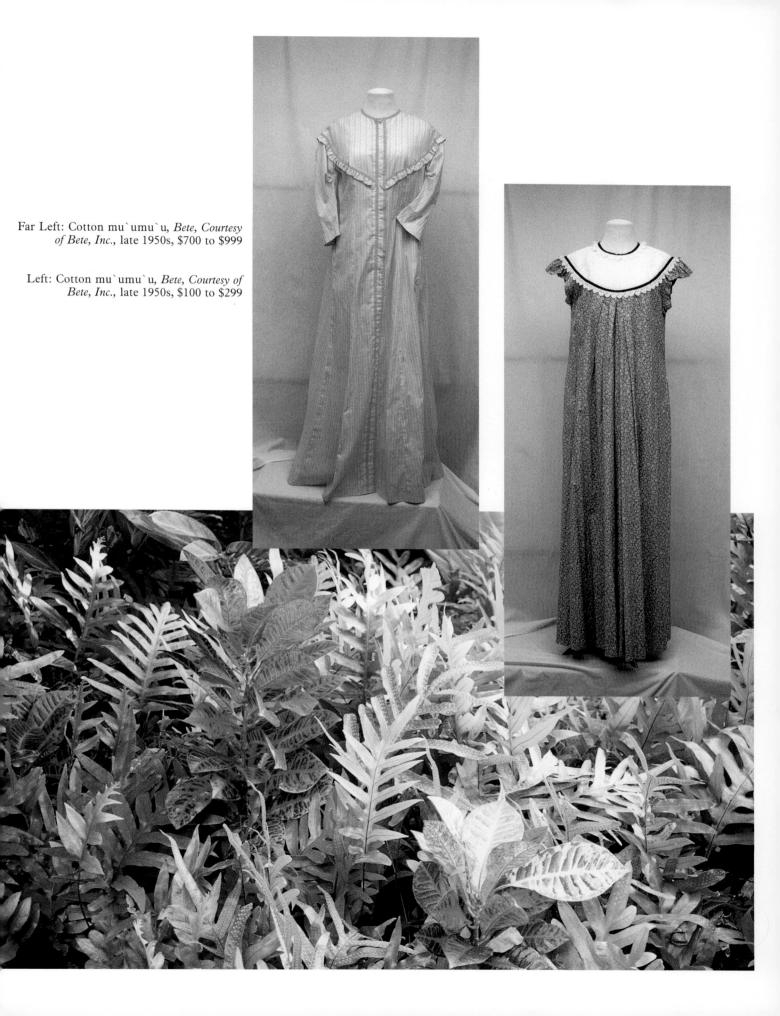

Far Left: Cotton mu`umu`u, *Bete, Courtesy of Bete, Inc.*, late 1950s, $700 to $999

Left: Cotton mu`umu`u, *Bete, Courtesy of Bete, Inc.*, late 1950s, $100 to $299

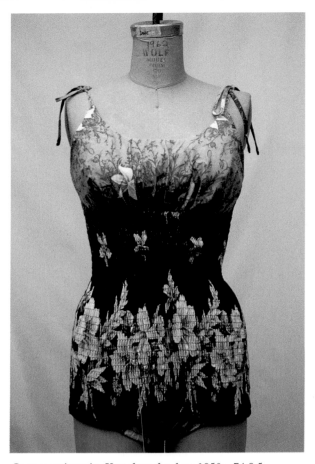

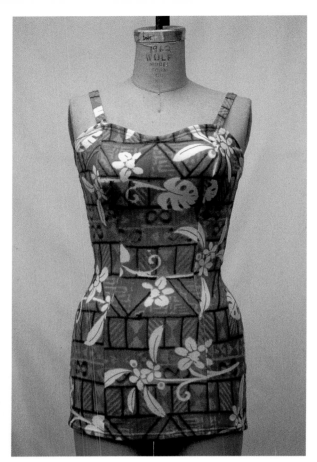

Cotton swimsuit, *Kamehameha,* late 1950s, 74.8.5, $100 to $299

Nylon swimsuit, *Kamehameha,* late 1950s, 86.8.186, $100 to $299

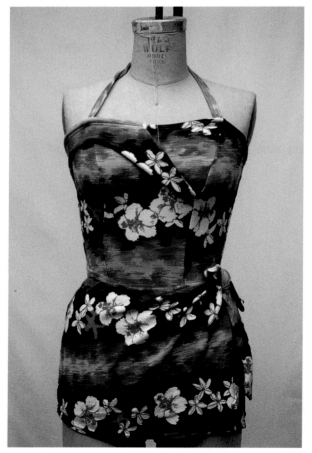

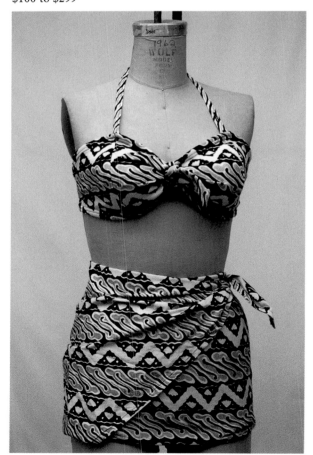

Nylon swimsuit, *Miss Hawaii by Kamehameha,* late 1950s, 98.15.3, $100 to $299

Nylon swimsuit, *Miss Hawaii by Kamehameha,* late 1950s, 98.15.4, $100 to $299

Men's Wear

In 1958, the Territorial Government agreed to "permit all its male employees to wear plain, short-sleeved sport shirts of subdued colors beginning on or about June 15 and extending through the end of Aloha Week. They will be required...to wear these shirts tucked in. Aloha shirt prints will not be permitted, but it is safe to assume that a conservative design on the pockets will be generally allowed." Iolani designed many shirts of this variety and became well known for conservatively styled aloha shirts, especially the jack shirt.

The conservative early 1960s were coming, and a new manufacturer –Reyns – came to fill the need for business shirts. Reyn McCullough had owned a men's clothing store in California before moving to Hawai`i. In 1959 he opened a men's shop then joined with Ruth Spooner to design preppy all-cotton aloha shirt with a button-down two-piece collar. McCullough carved out a niche in the local market by making an aloha shirt dignified enough for his local customers to wear for a casual evening out.

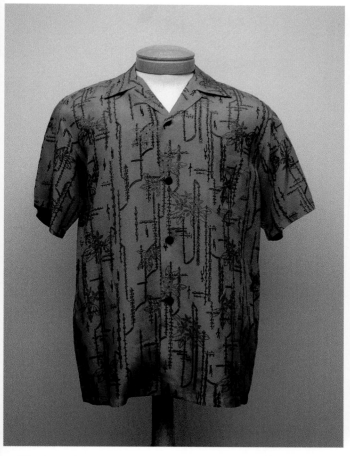

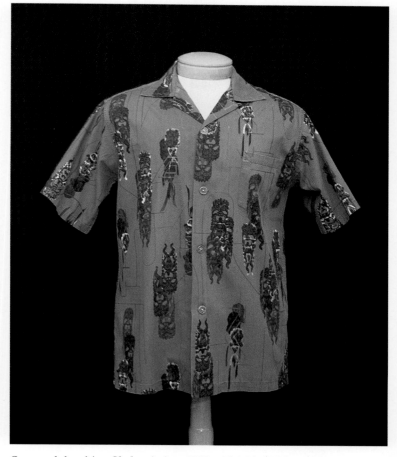

Silk aloha shirt, *Malihini*, fabric by *Shaheen's*, late 1950s, 73.1.4, $700 to $999

Cotton aloha shirt, *Shaheen's*, late 1950s, 95.2.12, $700 to $999

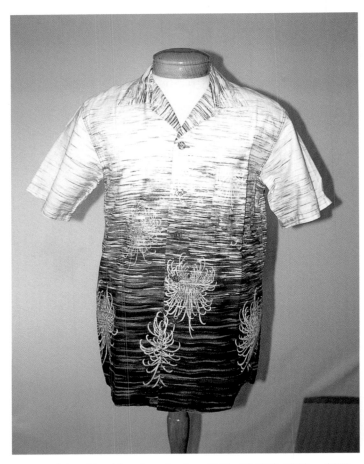

Cotton aloha shirt, *Kamehameha*, late 1950s, 76.27.9, $700 to $999

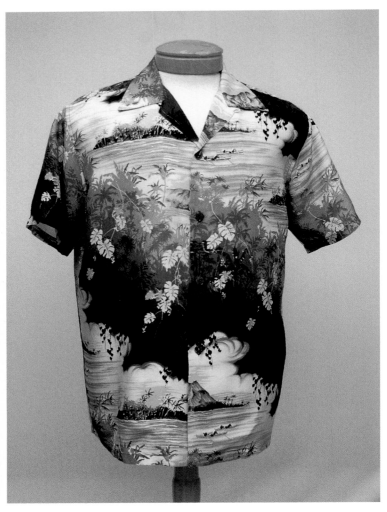

Silk aloha shirt, *Malihini, Made in Hawaii*, late 1950s, 76.27.13, $700 to $999

Cotton aloha shirt, custom made of yardage by *Shaheen's*, late 1950s, 94.2.5, $700 to $999

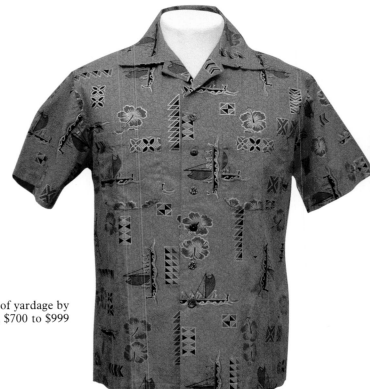

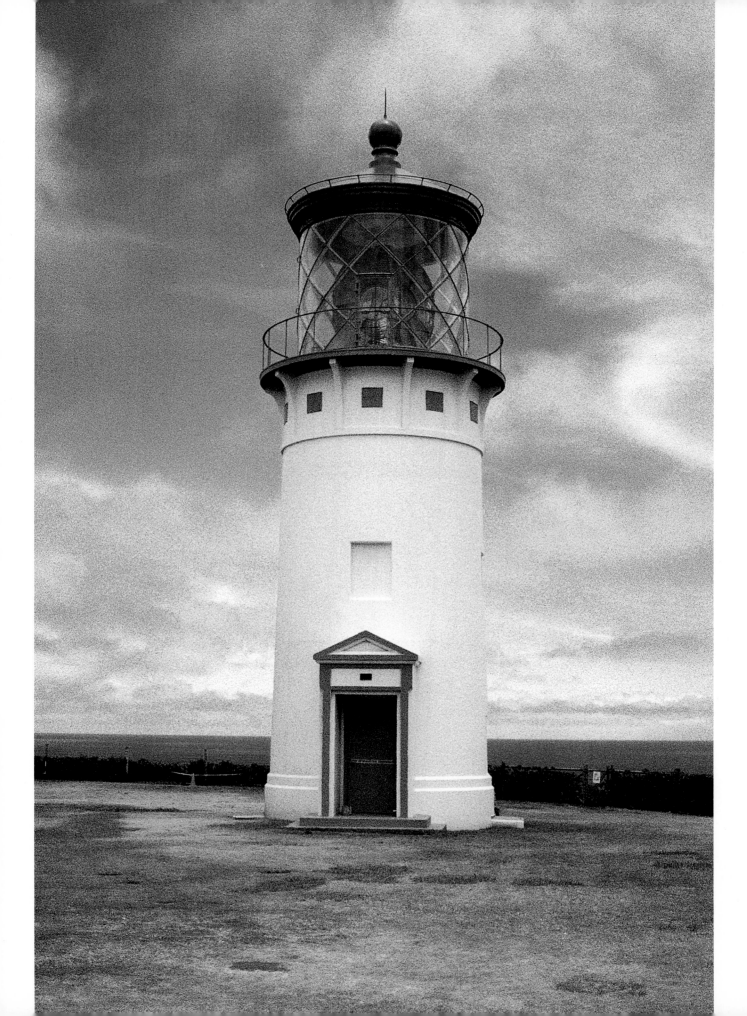

7. The 1960s
Aftermath Of Statehood

Cultural Context

After statehood, it was clear that there was a reciprocal relationship between Hawai`i and the mainland. Movies continued to be made about Hawai`i, and began to focus on surfing, historically the sport of Hawaiian kings. This sport became popular on the mainland as a result of the passion with which it was accepted by visitors to Hawai`i, particularly the military and tourists. As they returned home to the mainland from Hawai`i, they brought both the sport of surfing, and its requisite aloha shirt, into focus in California. The aloha shirt became associated in California with being a young, hip male, and wearing Hawaiian shirts in California high schools and colleges became a fad. At the same time as Hawai`i had an impact on the mainland, the State of Hawai`i focused on becoming even more Americanized - at least visually.

In terms of dress, while clothing imported from the mainland became even more popular, aloha attire began to resemble American clothing styles as well, while it continued to be used for Aloha Fridays, celebrations and dressy events. Aloha attire was manufactured and sold through American catalog companies, notably Sears, Montgomery Wards and JC Penneys. The conservatism of the early 1960s on the mainland was readily accepted in Hawai`i which was still rather conventional. When mainland trends shifted from the staid conservatism of the 1950s toward progressive liberalism and the social rebellions that fomented in the 1970s, Hawai`i did not follow along. Trends had often been slow to come to Hawai`i and in the 1960s Hawai`i did not eagerly embrace America's passion for the youth movement, pop art, rock and roll. This was apparent in the clothing of the 1960s in Hawai`i, as it is not until the very end of the 1960s that aloha attire begins to sport the wild fabrics that were famous on the mainland.

In 1962 The Hawaiian Fashion Guild staged 'Operation Liberation' in an attempt to encourage acceptance of printed aloha wear for business attire. The Guild gave each member of the State House of Representatives and Senate two aloha shirts. Mu`umu`u were presented to the women. As a result a Senate resolution was passed urging the regular use of aloha attire from Lei Day (May Day) throughout the summer. The Hawai`i Fashion Guild (an association of manufacturers) launched a campaign to institute Aloha Friday within the business community, encouraging employers to allow aloha attire to be worn to work every Friday. Aloha Friday officially commenced in 1966 with Willie Cannon, the President of the Bank of Hawai`i wearing aloha shirts to the office.[66] By the end of the decade the aloha shirt and

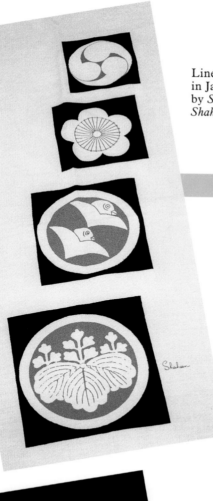

Linen-rayon blend engineered panel in Japanese mon (family crest) design by *Shaheen's, Courtesy of Camille Shaheen-Tunberg.* 1960s.

mu`umu`u had become a common sight in the office. At the same time surfers and tourists (who primarily came from the mainland US) took aloha shirts back to the mainland where the wearing of aloha shirts became a fad among young men, and led to a more casual style of dress overall. Herb Kawainui Kane noted, "By the late 1960s, informality of dress became something of a civil right."[67] Eventually, those young men ended up in positions of power in California and were able to push for a more casual style of dress in California offices, at least on Fridays. As a consequence, today's Casual Fridays in American corporations began as an offshoot of Hawaii's Aloha Fridays. It continues to spread internationally to Europe and Japan.

Fabrics

From the late 1950s on through the 1960s, hand screened fabrics were popular in Hawai`i, and these were produced by several firms, most of which were quite small. As noted by Gunter Von Hamm, (Von Hamm Textiles) solid colored linen and linen blend fabrics were favorite fabrics in the 1960s. Shaheen used these blends for engineered designs on vertical panels generally used down the front of women's dresses and mu`umu`u. The fabrics seen in aloha attire in the early 1960s tended to favor subtle designs; by the end of the decade the designs began to be much more bold. Kamehameha Garment Company produced stretch fabrics with Hawaiian prints on a nylon knit for swimsuit use in the early 1960s. In men's wear, the major innovation of the 1960s was the use of reverse prints in aloha shirts. Often called 'inside out shirts', the back side of the fabric was intentionally used as the right side of the fabric on aloha shirts.

Linen-rayon blend engineered panel in fisherman design by *Shaheen's, Courtesy of Camille Shaheen-Tunberg.* 1960s.

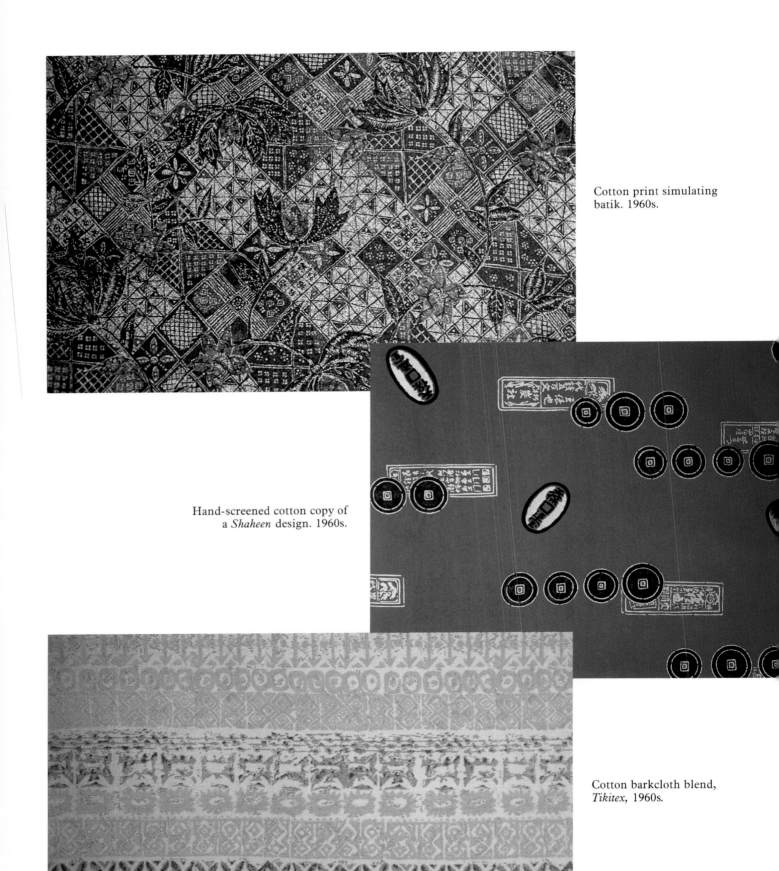

Cotton print simulating
batik. 1960s.

Hand-screened cotton copy of
a *Shaheen* design. 1960s.

Cotton barkcloth blend,
Tikitex, 1960s.

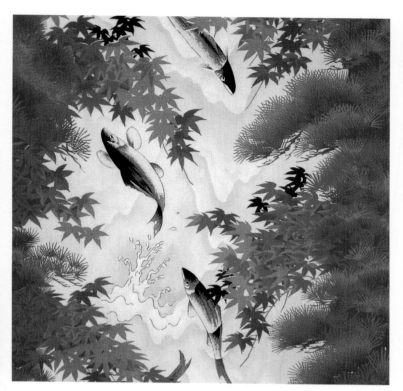

Cotton, Japanese fish design, 1960s.

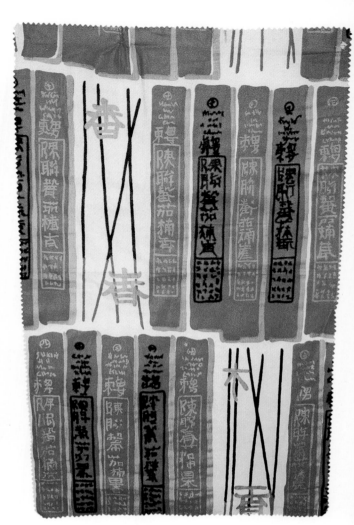

Linen blend; *Shaheen's* engineered panel; Japanese mon design. *Courtesy of Camille Shaheen-Tunberg,* 1960s.

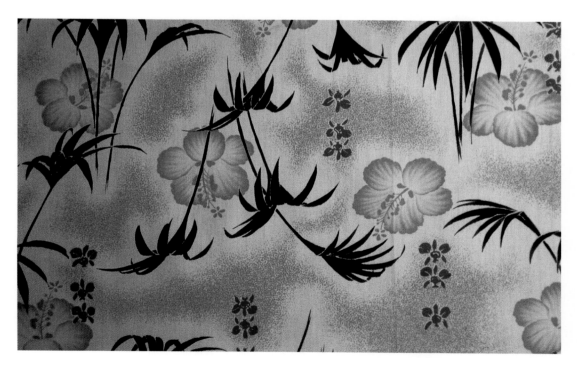

Cotton blend, *Pacific Sportswear,* 1960s

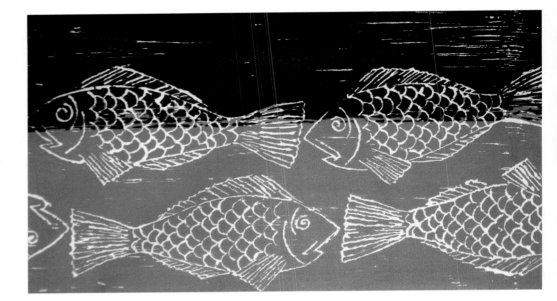

Cotton fabric, screen printed in Makaha, Hawaii. *Hawaiian Textiles* by Gunter Von Hamm, 1960s

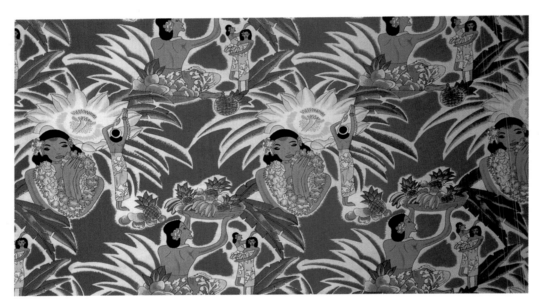

Cotton blend; recoloration of original Matson Menu design. 1960s.

Cotton, volcano tapa design. 1960s.

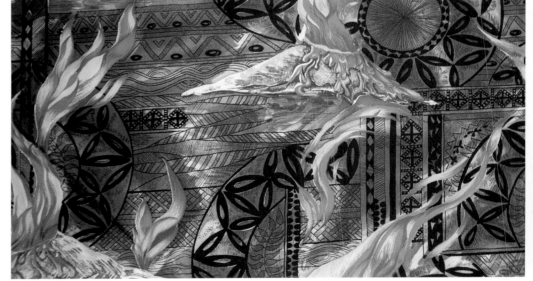

Clothing Production

The post-statehood boom especially benefited the fashion industry. Mens wear manufacturers diversified with various swimshorts and baggy shorts called Jams® to meet surfer's demands. (The term Jams® is a copyrighted name owned by the inventor, David Rochlen).[68] Two new kinds of jackets were invented. Kona jackets, inspired by the need for protection from winds on the Kona side of the Big Island, were Hawaiian print-lined windbreakers of translucent nylon. For a more formal look, tailored sport jackets of Hawaiian print fabrics, were designed in Hawai`i and custom made in Hong Kong. These jackets were especially favored by entertainers. By the end of the sixties, eighty-five firms were ringing up a wholesale volume of $34 million in annual sales. In addition to producing aloha attire, the Hawaiian garment manufacturers produced a great deal of non-Hawaiian clothing, but often with Hawaiian prints. Kamehameha's trademark during the 1960s was brightly colored designs and the company was known for its brightly colored print shirts, dresses, mu`umu`u, holomu`u and sun suits. Because the company was one of the original sponsors of the Miss Hawai`i contest, Kamehameha produced a line of swimwear under the Miss Hawai`i label; contestants for the title of Miss Hawai`i frequently modeled new designs in mainland shows. Hawaiian swimsuit designs thus had an impact on mainland swimwear.[69]

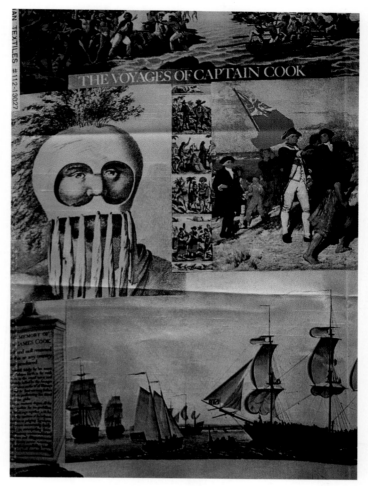

Nylon photo print, 1960s

Hilo Hattie, a large tourist-oriented fashion business that sells mu`umu`u, aloha shirts, and other garments originated in Hilo (on the Big Island) in 1963. The company was named after a famous Hawaiian entertainer who performed in numerous clubs both in Hawai`i and on the mainland between the late 1930s and her retirement in 1969. This company has consistently focused on the production of aloha attire for the tourist market.

Women's Attire

In Hawai`i, the mu`umu`u consistently increased in popularity during the 1960s. The popularity of this dress at home was spurred on by its being in vogue on the US mainland. Due to tourism and President Kennedy's vow to support the American fashion industry, mu`umu`u became popular on the mainland at all socio-economic levels. The First Lady had a black velvet mu`umu`u made for her by the Hawaiian designer, Bete, and other celebrity women had splendid holoku and mu`umu`u designed for them as well.

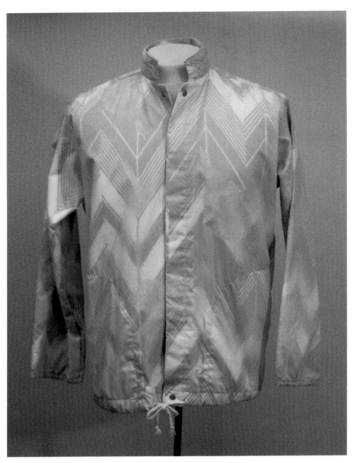

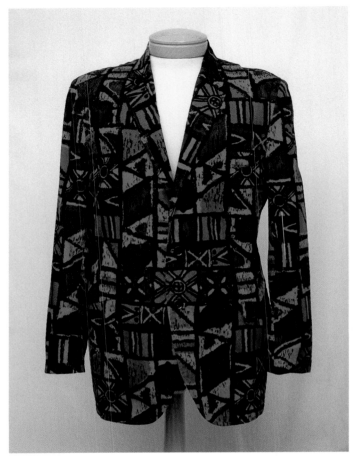

Nylon over cotton, Kona jacket, *Hawaiian Holiday*, 1960s, 85.14.5, $100 to $299

Cotton sportscoat, *Tailored in Hong Kong*, 1960s, 95.7.1, $100 to $299

Fashion influence to and from Hawai`i has been reciprocal since the 1960s. American and European fashions had a dramatic impact on Hawaiian apparel during this decade. The slender fitting sheath of western fashion was incorporated into the Hawaiian holoku and the mu`umu`u. Because of its simple lines, the sheath-styled holoku had little in the way of applied details; its beauty derives from the simple flowing lines and the use of elegant fabrics. Mu`umu`u were worn short, sometimes as short as mid-thigh, and were simply designed with bold Hawaiian prints. As mu`umu`u were the hot fashion item of the 1960s, less holomu`u were produced in the 1960s. Because holoku were now considered formal evening garments, dress fabrics such as lace, velvet, satin and silk were used. Lace became extremely popular, especially for wedding holoku. By the 1960s, Hawaiian fabrics were only found in mu`umu`u, holomu`u, and aloha shirts, but no longer appeared in holoku. Hawaiian fabrics were considered casual by then and therefore more appropriate for daytime wear.

A women's wear manufacturer, Princess Kaiulani was started in 1961 with the intention of making mu`umu`u more elegant. Joan Anderson wanted to design mu`umu`u that were more flattering to the figure; she preferred subdued prints and fabrics. Anderson started adding touches of lace, ribbons, and ruffles. Non-traditional fabrics, such as English chintz, were used for the slim styles. Named after the last Princess of the Hawaiian monarchy, this company focuses on Victorian and Edwardian styles for their holoku, holomu`u and mu`umu`u.

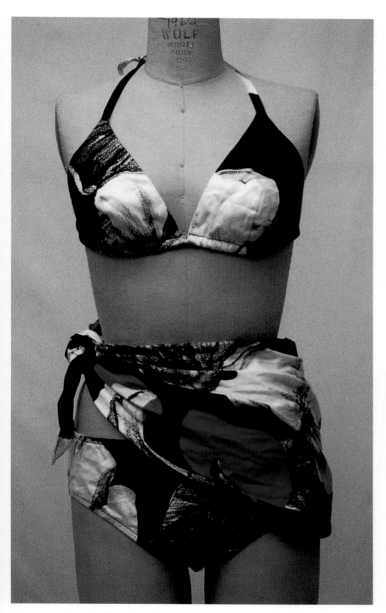

Cotton swimsuit, *Kamehameha*, 1960s, 86.8.189, under $100

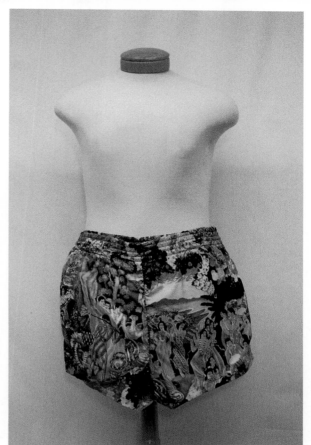

Nylon swim trunks in Matson Menu design, 1960s, *Kamehameha, Courtesy of Kamehameha Garment Co.*, $100 to $299

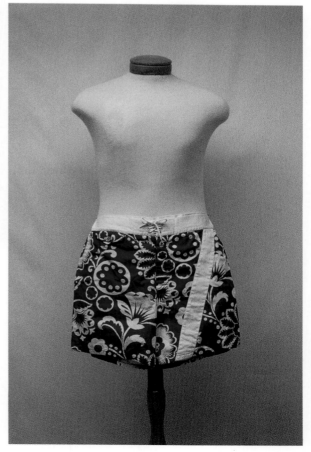

Cotton board shorts, *Kamehameha*, 1960s, 86.8.299, $100 to $299

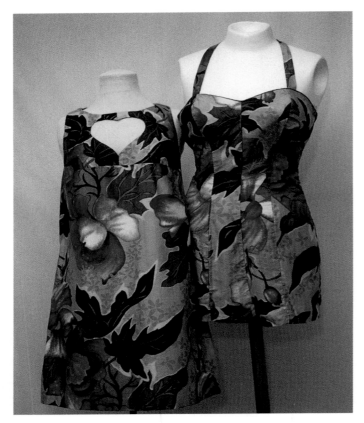

Cotton swimsuit and cover-up, *Kamehameha*, 1960s , 86.8.193, $100 to $299

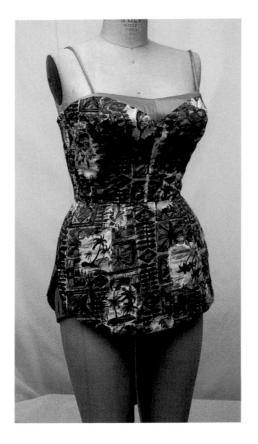

Cotton bikini set, *Kamehameha*, 1960s, 88.8.124, under $100

Cotton swimsuit, *Kamehameha*, 1960s , 86.8.193, under $100

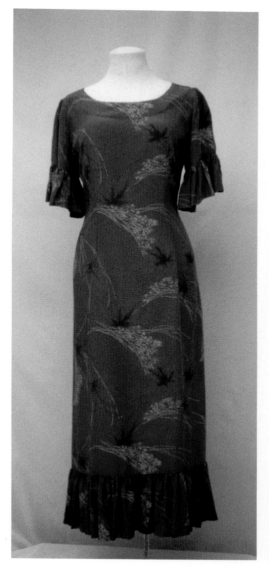

Silk holomuʻu, custom made, 1960s , 98.17.3, $300 to $699

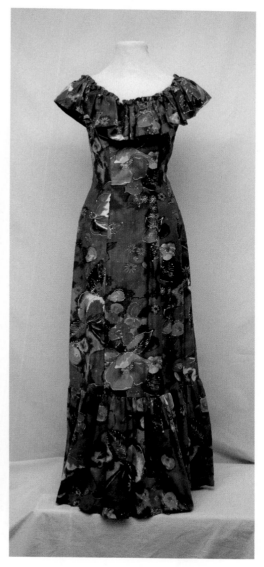

Cotton sateen holomuʻu, *Lauhala* 1960s, 87.9.1, $300 to $699

By the 1960s, aloha attire was well accepted not only for Aloha Fridays, but was considered particularly appropriate for special events such as Aloha Week. Mrs. Mildred Briner, from Kamehameha Garment Company suggested in 1961 that:

Island women attending Aloha Week activities will be appropriately attired if they're wearing colorful, Hawaiʻi-made clothes and flowers in their hair. For the King and Queen's reception ... wear holoku and holomuʻu to complement the 1880 period attire of the royal couple. For church services ...conservative holomuʻu, shell leis, lauhala hats trimmed with feather or flower leis, with accessories suitable for a dressy ensemble. For the Royal Ball - glamorous holoku, formal gowns to complement the Queen's white taffeta gown, copied from one worn by Kapio-lani before the turn of the century. For [musical] events at the Waikiki Shell- sundresses that can double for cocktail wear, sweaters and island-made sandals.[70]

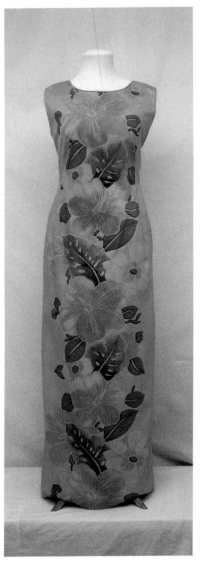

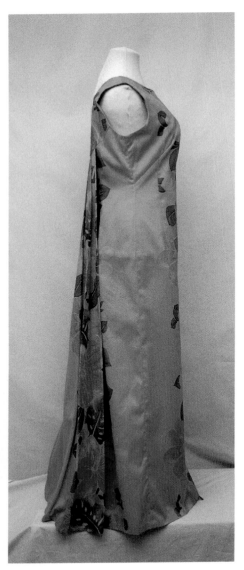

Acrylic holomu`u, custom made,
1960s, 89.10.2, $300 to $699

Side view, acrylic holomu`u, 1960s,
89.10.2, $300 to $699

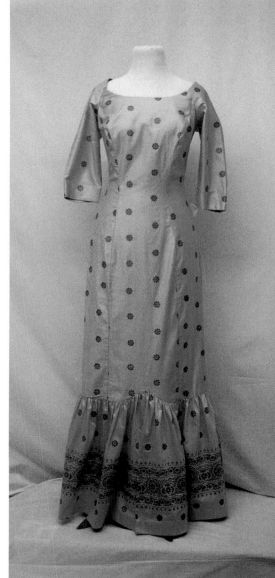

Cotton sateen holomu`u, *Kamehameha*, 1960s,
86.8.48, $300 to $699

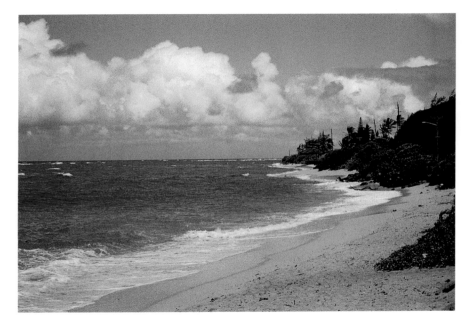

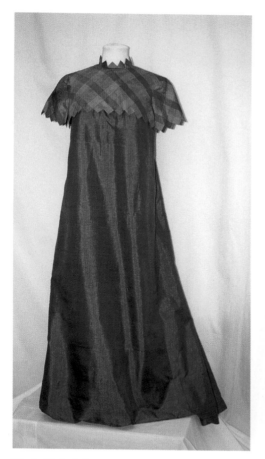

Thai silk holoku, custom made, 1960s, 97.10.1 $300 to $699

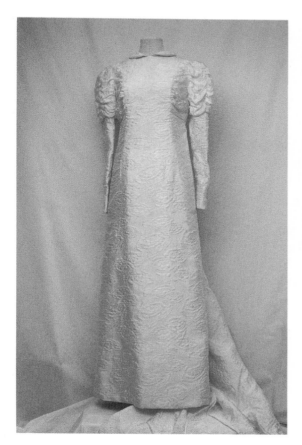

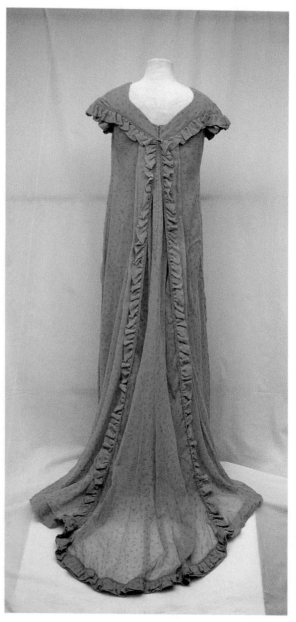

Cotton voile holoku, *"Huapala"* designed by *Bete* for Queen Elizabeth, *Courtesy of Bete, Inc.* 1960s, $700 to $999

Polyester brocade holoku, custom made, 1960s, 74.7.3, $300 to $699

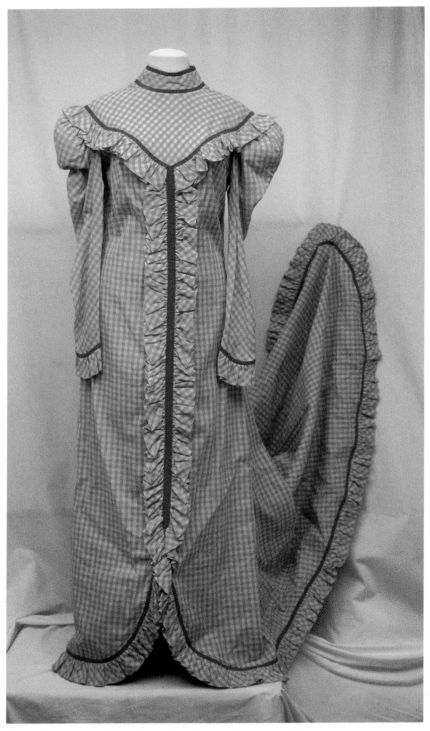

Cotton holoku, "Kaialani and Emmalani" designed by *Bete, Courtesy of Bete, Inc.*, 1960s, $300 to $699

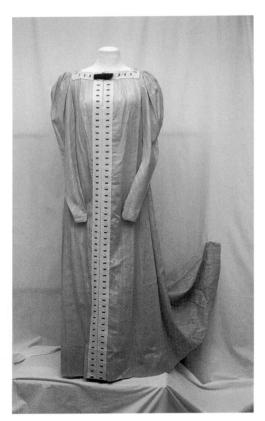

Cotton holoku, *"Hanohano"* designed by *Bete, Courtesy of Bete, Inc.*, 1960s, $100 to $299

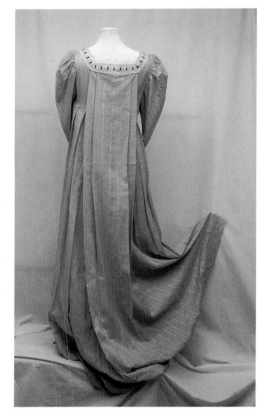

Cotton holoku, *"Hanohano"* designed by *Bete, Courtesy of Bete, Inc.*, 1960s, $100 to $299

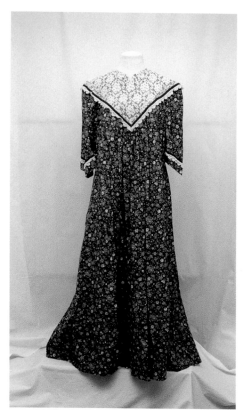

Cotton mu`umu`u, designed by *Bete*,
Courtesy of Bete, Inc., 1960s, $100 to $299

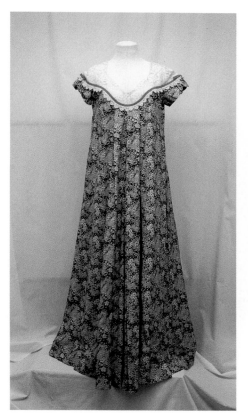

Cotton mu`umu`u, *"Liliuokalani"*
designed by *Bete*, *Courtesy of Bete, Inc.*,
1960s, $100 to $299

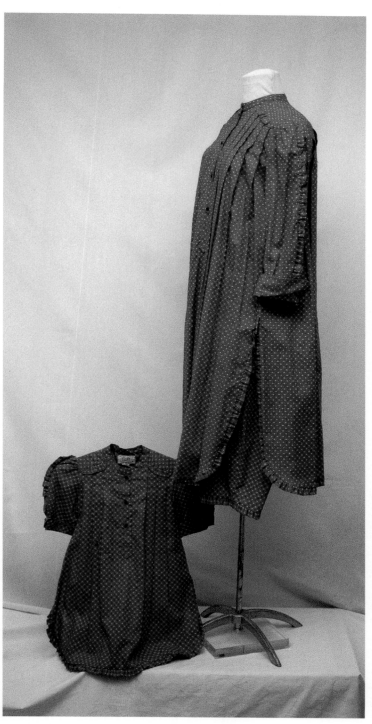

Cotton calico mu`umu`u, *"New Englander"* (mother and daughter
set), by *Bete Inc.* 1960s, 81.1.3, $100 to $299

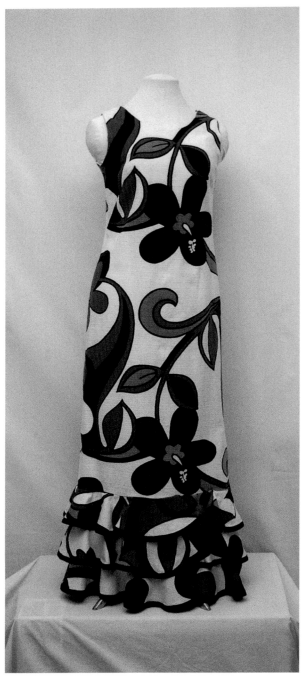

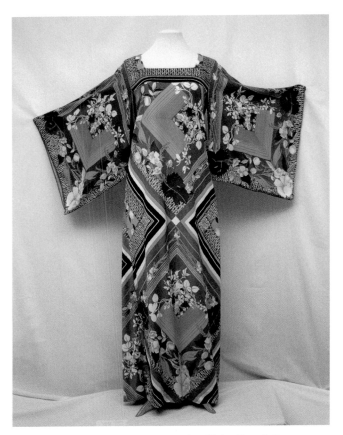

Nylon mu`umu`u, *Jane M;* worn by Claire Booth Luce, 1960s, 79.11.2, $300 to $699

Cotton barkcloth mu`umu`u, *Malihini*, 1960s , 84.20.18, $700 to $999

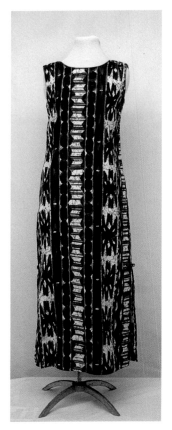

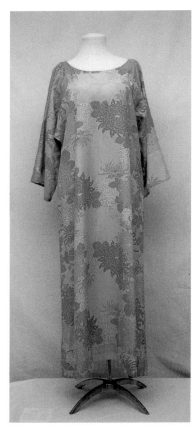

Cotton mu`umu`u, *Tropicana*, 1960s , 84.20.12, $100 to $299

Silk mu`umu`u, *Hata Dry Goods, Hilo*, 1960s , 82.14.9, $100 to $299

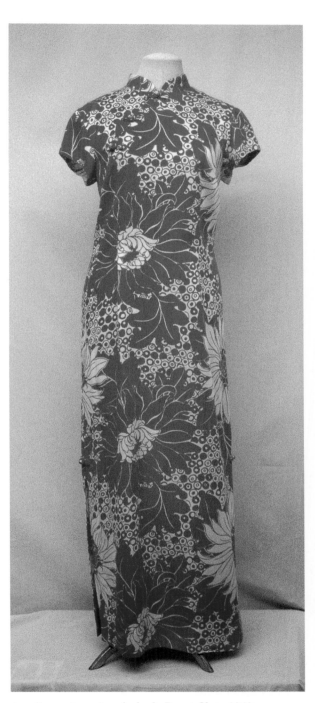

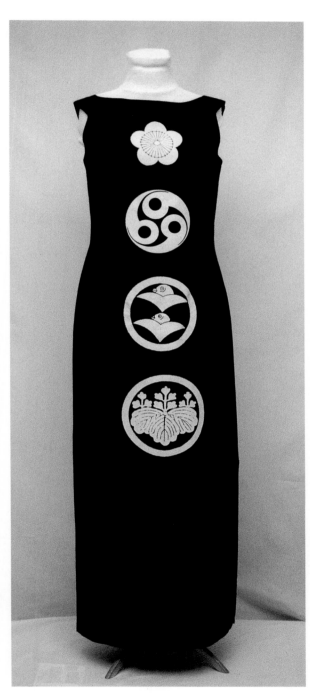

Acrylic mu`umu`u, *Andrade Resort Shops*,1960s,
76.29.27, $300 to $699

Cotton mu`umu`u, *Alfred Shaheen*, 1960s , 84.21.26,
$300 to $699

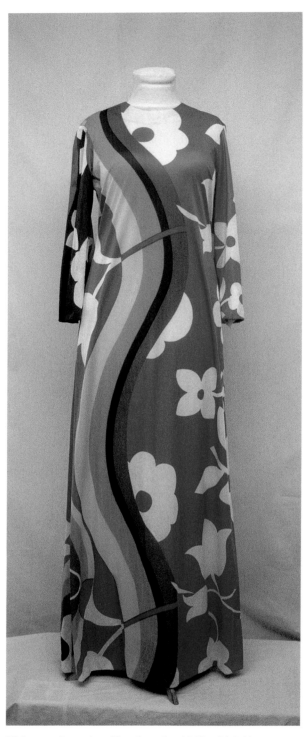

Nylon mu`umu`u, *Kamehameha*, 1960s, 86.8.42,
$300 to $699

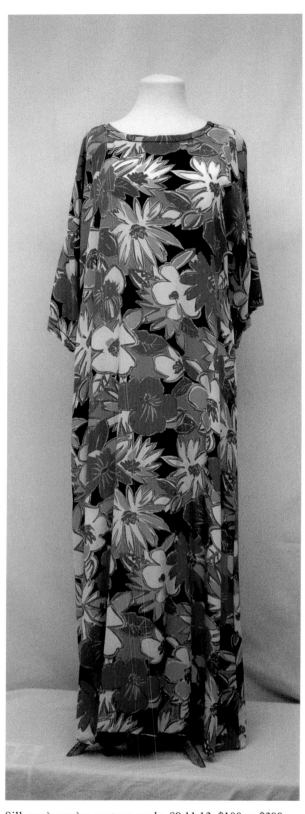

Silk mu`umu`u, custom made, 89.11.12, $100 to $299

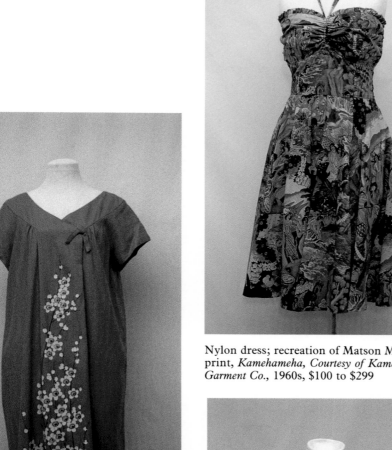

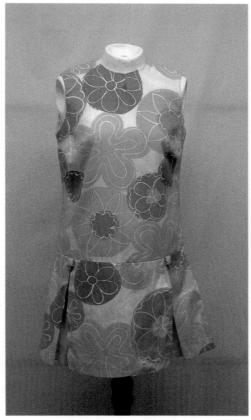

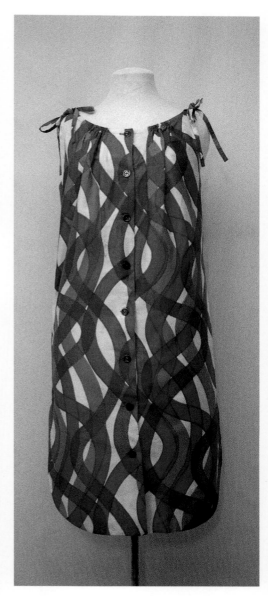

Nylon dress; recreation of Matson Menu print, *Kamehameha, Courtesy of Kamehameha Garment Co.,* 1960s, $100 to $299

en mu`umu`u, *Arawaka's* , 1960s, 17.7, $100 to $299

Cotton sateen mu`umu`u, *Kamehameha.* 1960s 86.8.49, $100 to $299

Cotton pique mu`umu`u, *Kamehameha,* 86.8.298, 60s, under $100

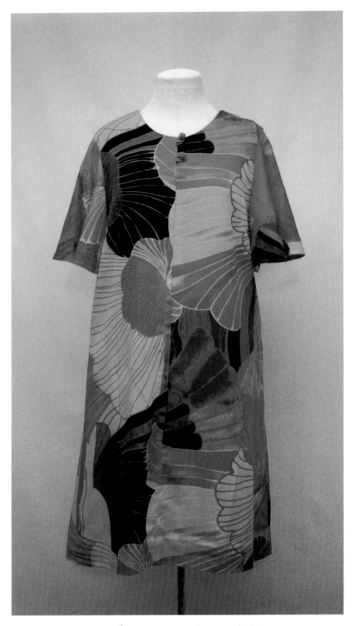

Acrylic mu`umu`u, Í960s. 98.14.8, $100 to $299

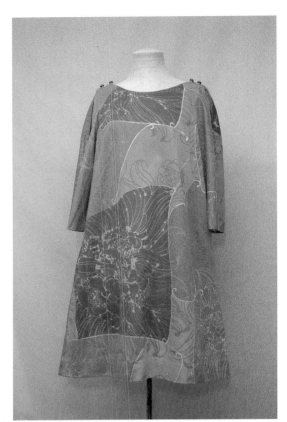

Acrylic mu`umu`u, *Waltah Clarke's*, 1960s, 87. 9.5, $100 to $299

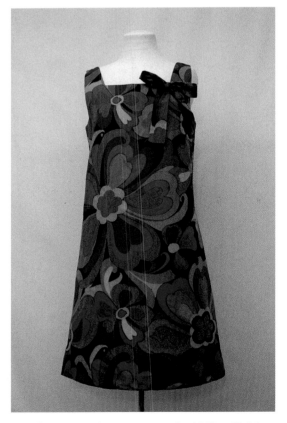

Acrylic mu`umu`u, custom made, 1960s , 98.9.1, $100 to $299

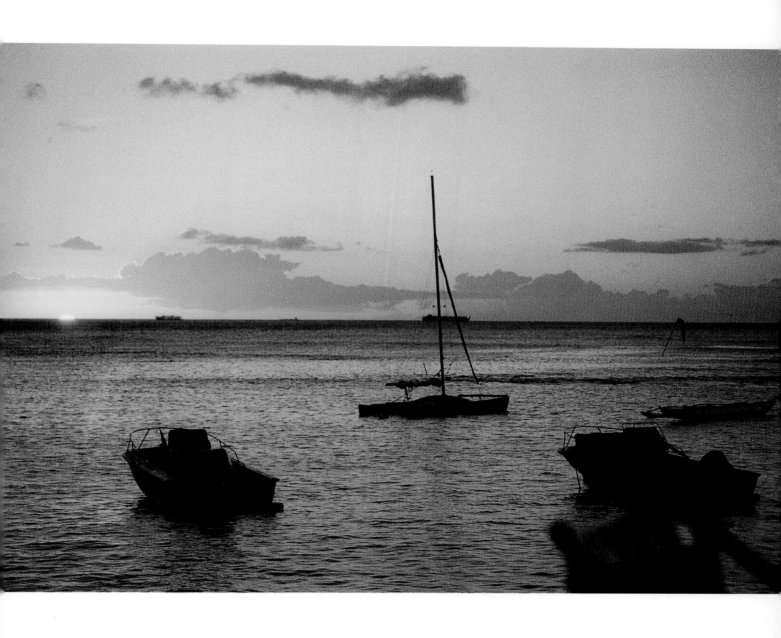

Men's Wear

In the early 1960s, short aloha shirts were in vogue, particularly the shirt called a 'jack shirt'. These were styled with the Eisenhower jacket in mind; they had button tabs at the shirt hem that hit between the waist and hip. Often manufactured in solid fabrics, the jack shirt with a small logo on the pocket was primarily worn by men who worked with the public. This may have been an outgrowth of the restrictions placed on aloha shirts for business use in the previous decade. Many islanders remember the jack shirt as being a uniform of sorts for men who worked in hotels, as a predecessor to aloha shirts worn as uniforms for those in service industries - what has become known as identity apparel. Identity apparel may have started in the late 1950s, but became popular in the 1960s when United Airlines started using aloha shirts and Hawaiian attire for its stewardesses.[71]

Reyn McCullough began his aloha shirt business by introducing a bit of tailoring to the aloha shirt; his shirts were made with the more formal two-piece collar construction and button down collars. Originally his shirts were all cotton. Reyn noticed that the most popular shirts were well worn and bleached out — this style was worn by surfers. McCullough decided to turn the fabric inside out in 1961 to simulate this look. By turning the brightly colored floral and calico prints inside out, he created a muted look that more nearly resembled the bleached out look worn by the surfers. One story claims that a Waikiki bartender named Pat Dorian asked Spooner to make the shirts with the fabric turned inside out. Whatever the inspiration, the effect was well received. Reversed print aloha shirts became extremely popular and are today worn by Hawaiian businessmen.[72]

In the 1960s, Hawaiian shirts became even more popular on the US mainland due to the impact of surfing culture in California. As surfers came to Hawai`i to surf the North Shore, they returned with aloha shirts and shorts; these had a significant impact on the American sportswear industry which readily copied Hawaiian styles. In addition to aloha shirts, California manufacturers copied Jams®, reverse print shirts, and kona jackets.

"The Guru of Surf Wear," David Rochlen began his factory in 1965 after relocating to Hawai`i from the mainland. He began by selling surfboards and included clothing in his store. Completely designing the garments, Rochlen even chose the print and color. His success with Jams® (a baggy swim short made with Hawaiian prints) is legendary. In 1978, referring to Ocean Pacific and other mainland firms that were producing adapted Hawaiian styles at a lower price, Rochlen commented, "I'm seeking à selective market. Me, I'm the Porsche, those others are Datsun." In the mid 1980s, Rochlen saw the big boom in the print market coming and for a year or two was the largest garment manufacturer in Hawai`i.[73] In addition to Jams®, the company produced Surf Line shirts that appealed to both the younger and the more mature consumers.[74]

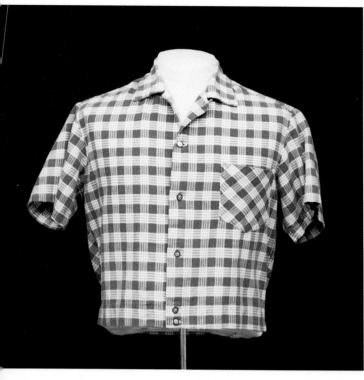

Palaka shirt, Jack shirt style *Andrade's*, 1960s 98.2.1, $100 to $299

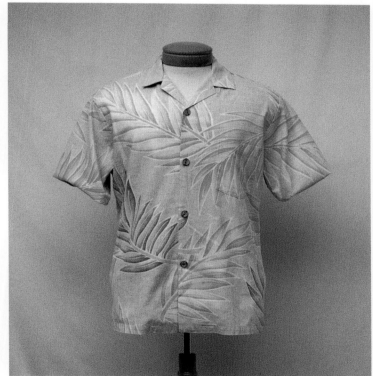

Cotton aloha shirt, *Surfline Hawaii*, 1960s, 98.17.12, $100 to $299

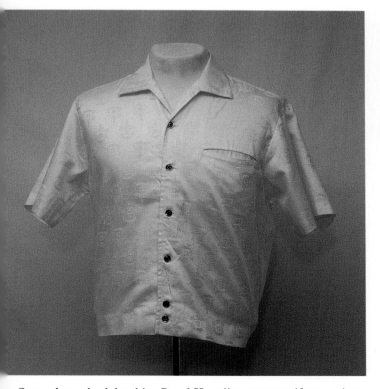

Cotton brocade aloha shirt, Royal Hawaiian crest motif woven into fabric. Jack shirt style *Kamehameha*, 1960s, 98.15.2, $300 to $699

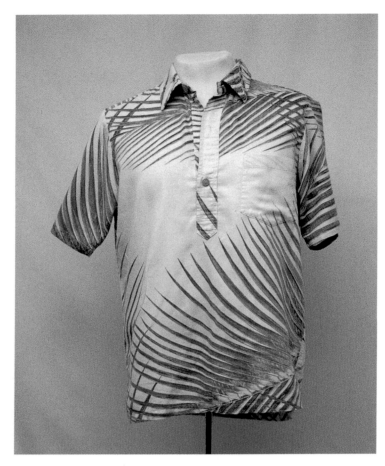

Cotton aloha shirt, *Ross Sutherland,*
1960s 98.17.10, $300 to $699

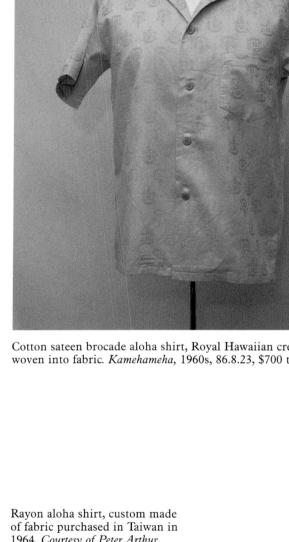

Cotton sateen brocade aloha shirt, Royal Hawaiian crest motif
woven into fabric. *Kamehameha,* 1960s, 86.8.23, $700 to $999

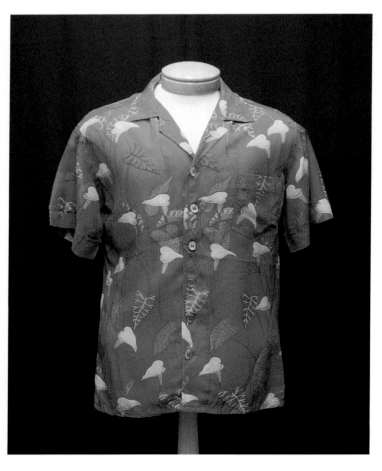

Rayon aloha shirt, custom made
of fabric purchased in Taiwan in
1964, *Courtesy of Peter Arthur,*
1960s, $300 to $699

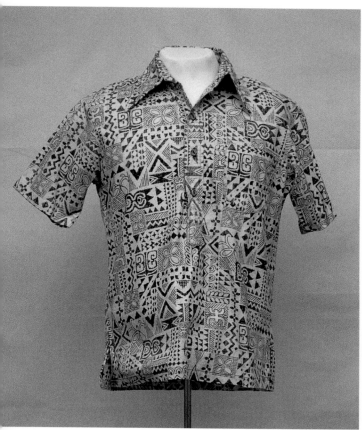

Cotton aloha shirt, *Holo Holo*,
1960s, 95.2.7, $100 to $299

Cotton aloha shirt, *Shaheen's, Courtesy of Camille Shaheen- Tunberg*,
1960s, $300 to $699

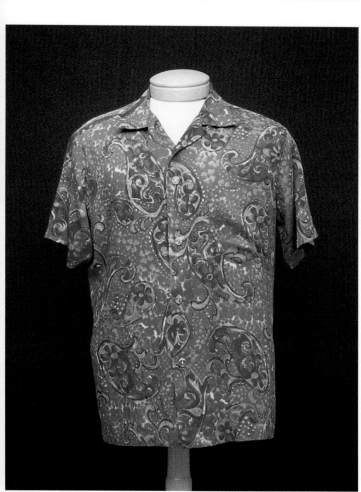

Silk aloha shirt, *Royal Hawaiian
Manufacturing Co.*, 1960s, 97.11.12,
$100 to $299

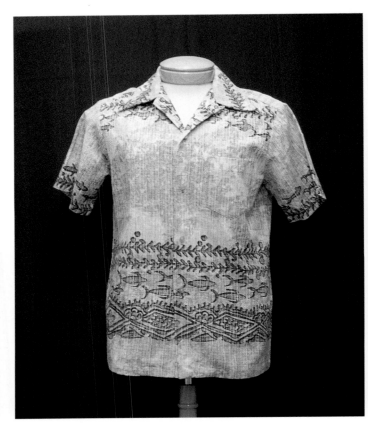

Cotton barkcloth aloha shirt, *Lehua,* 1960s , 99.1.7, $100 to $299

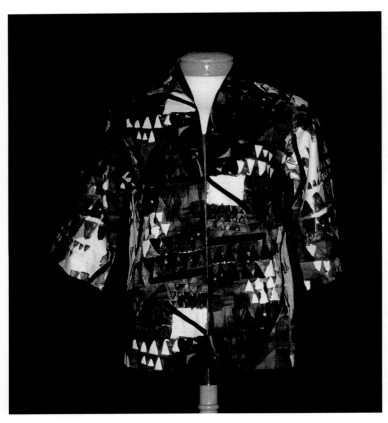

Cotton barkcloth aloha shirt — *Kamehameha* copy of a *Shaheen* shirt. Alfred Shaheen introduced the 3/4 sleeve as a dressier aloha shirt. 1960s, 99.1.8, $100 to $299

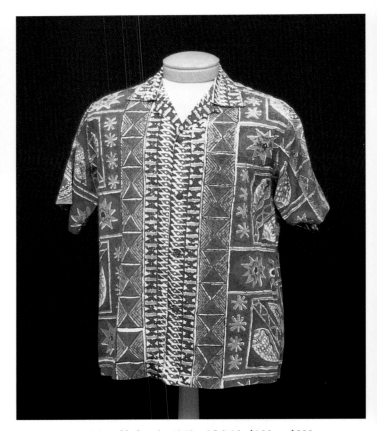

Cotton aloha shirt, *Shaheen's,* 1960s, 95.2.10, $100 to $299

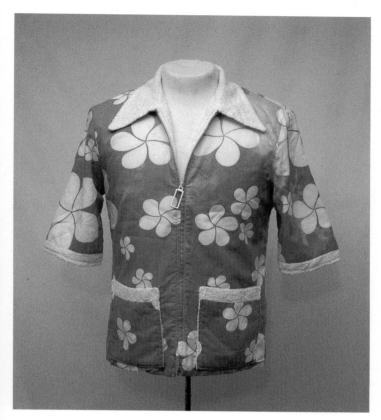

Cotton and terry cloth beach jacket, *Mauna Kea*, late 1960s, 98.13.7, $100 to $299

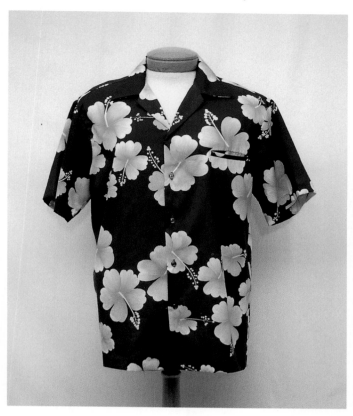

Polyester aloha shirt, *Hilo Hattie*, *Courtesy* of *Hilo Hattie*, late 1960s, under $100

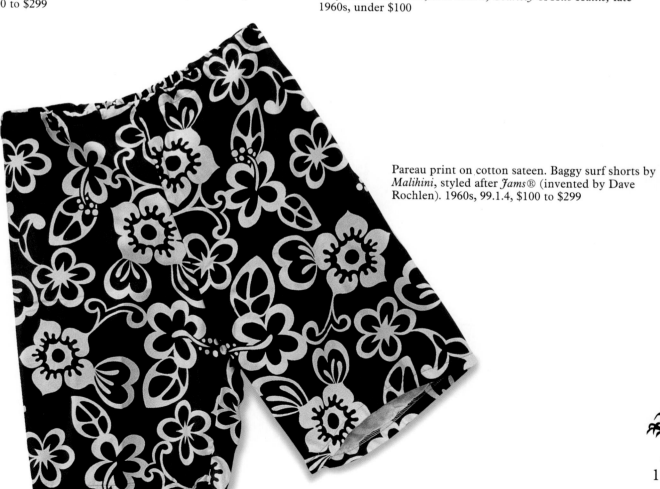

Pareau print on cotton sateen. Baggy surf shorts by *Malihini*, styled after *Jams*® (invented by Dave Rochlen). 1960s, 99.1.4, $100 to $299

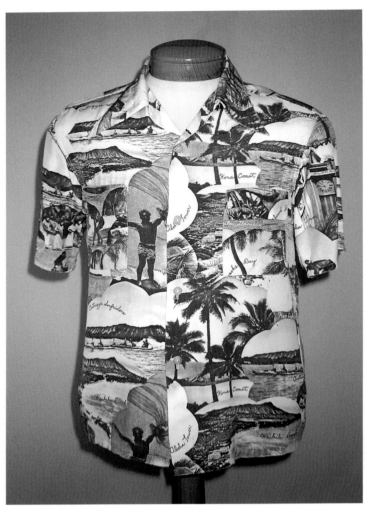

Rayon aloha shirt, late 1960s, $700 to $999

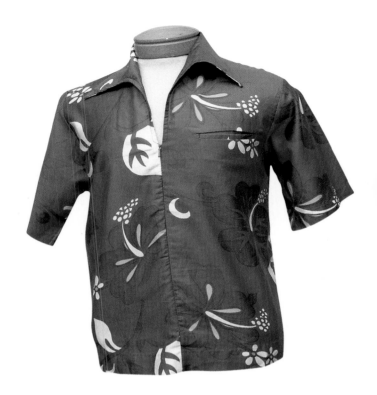

Cotton sateen aloha shirt, *Kamehameha*, 1960s, 86.8.21, $300 to $699

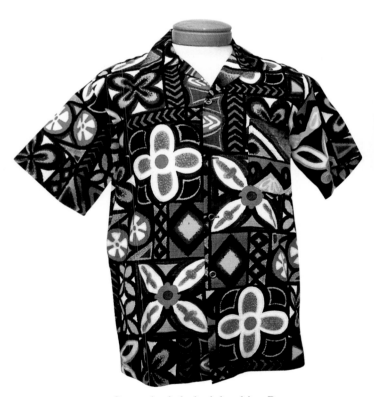

Cotton barkcloth aloha shirt, *Pomare*, late 1960s, 97.6.2, $300 to $699

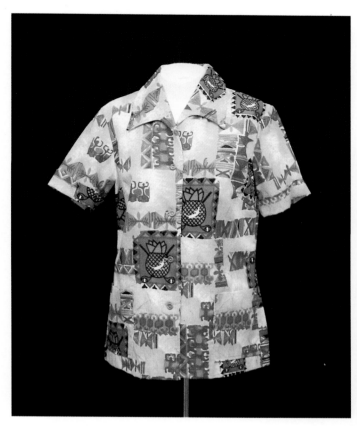

Cotton/polyester blend aloha shirt for women, *Keone*, late 1960s
77.11.18, $100 to $299

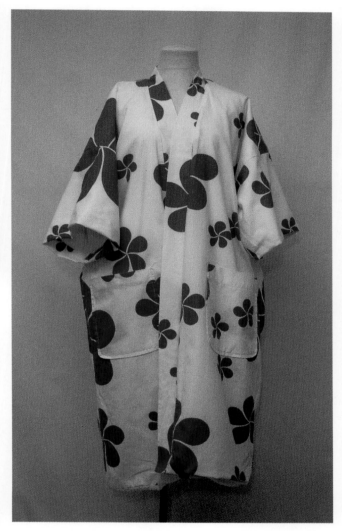

Cotton broadcloth and terry cloth, *Mauna Kea*. Women's
beach cover-up, late 1960s , 98.13.6, $100 to $299

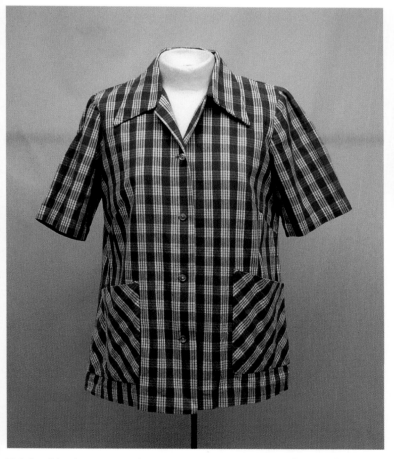

Palaka shirt for women. *Arakawas.*, late 1960s, 98.19.1, $100 to $299

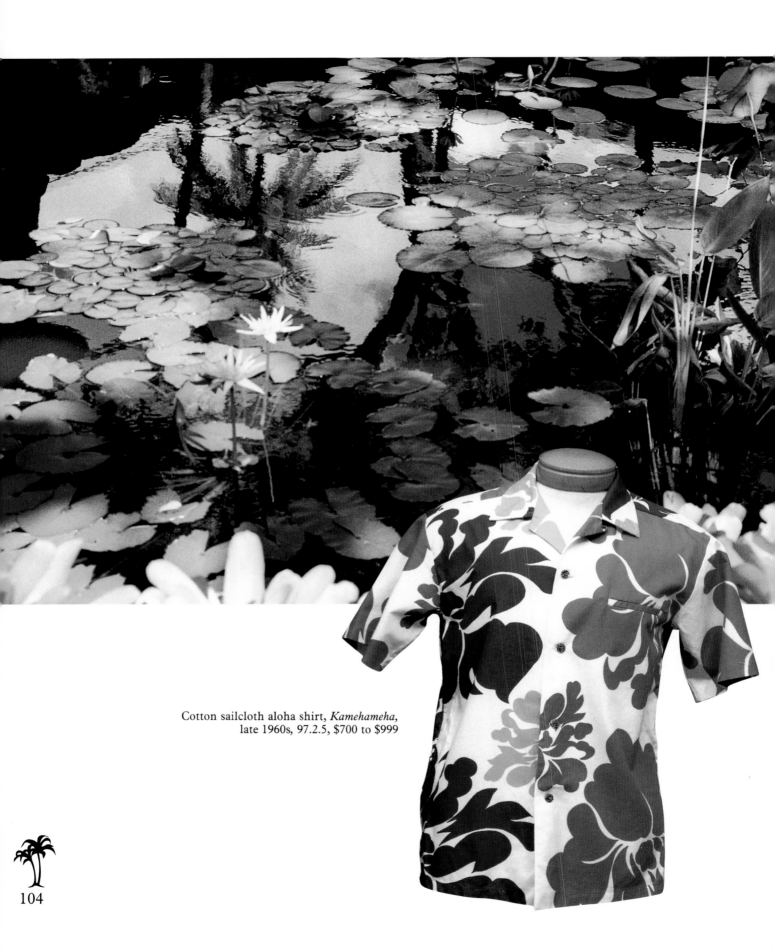

Cotton sailcloth aloha shirt, *Kamehameha*,
late 1960s, 97.2.5, $700 to $999

8. The 1970s
Ethnic Celebration

Cultural Context

All over America in the 1970s, we were fascinated by ethnicity and focused on it in numerous ways. People "got in touch" with their ethnic origins, and discovered the beauty of traditional arts and crafts from cultures all over the world. The celebration of ethnic difference was seen in clothing as well as other forms of material culture. For the previous decade, aloha attire looked like American dress with Hawaiian fabrics; in the late 1970s the Hawaiian garment designers drew their inspiration from all over the globe.

Culture continued as an integrating idea throughout this decade, and remains the focal point in Hawai`i at the end of this century. In the latter half of the 1970s Hawai`i refocused on its own cultural history. There was a new attention paid to the traditional crafts and practices of Hawaiian culture. The Hokule`a, a replica of the early Hawaiian voyaging canoes, had its first long-distance voyage in 1975. This stimulated Hawaiian imaginations and led to a resurgence in Hawaiian craft production which set the stage for what would be termed "The Hawaiian Renaissance," the focus of the next chapter.

Fabrics

Celebration of cultural diversity in aloha attire went beyond the incorporation of design details from other cultures, to wholesale adoption of fabrics from other cultures. Batik fabrics from Indonesia were very popular in aloha shirts and mu`umu`u, kente cloth, dashiki prints and batiks from Africa were used in mu`umu`u. Chinese brocades and Thai silks were popular in holoku as well as silk blend fabrics that simulated the Philippines' traditional piña cloth made from pineapple fiber. These fabrics were used in all forms of aloha attire in the early 1970s. By the late 1970s, as Hawai`i began to rediscover its material culture, traditional Hawaiian designs returned to aloha wear, done on both rayon's and synthetics. Cottons once again were fashionable. While design lines and styles followed western fashion, the fabrics were uniquely Hawaiian, tapa prints and tropical motifs in very bold color combinations were favored.

Clothing Production

Aloha attire production increased by the end of the 1970s. The current owner of Malihini found that there was a huge amount of business in aloha attire in the Hawaiian Islands after 1976. She remem-

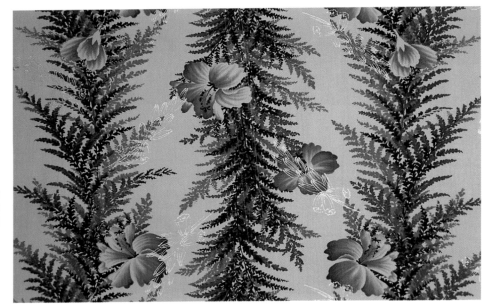

Cotton with metallic paint:
Reef Sportswear copy of a
Shaheen design

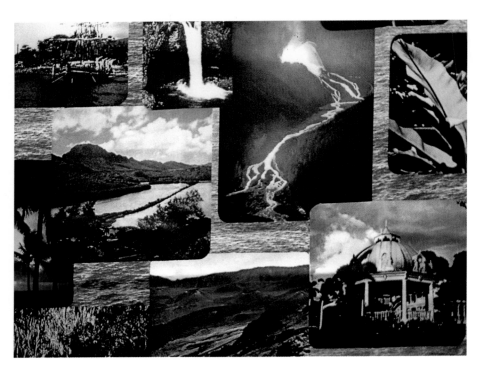

Nylon photo print

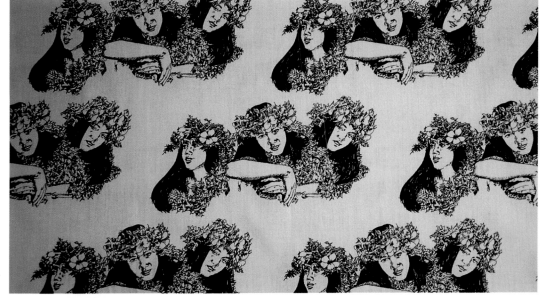

Cotton screen print, *Alan Akina*

bered traveling to the Neighbor Islands once every two months, spending an entire week on each island. "That's how much business there was," she said. That was the heyday when mainland tourists were Hawaii's — and Malihini's — mainstay. Annual sales for the company at that time were around $5 million.[75]

> Colorful Hawaiian prints from territorial days are being used not only for men's aloha shirts but for women's blouses, jackets, dresses and shorts as well. Imprinted with island motifs - pineapples, surfers, tropical flowers, hula girls, ukuleles, steamships and coconut palms - silkies are executed in the art deco style.... Renewed popularity began, not with designers, but with surfers who began to buy old forties shirts in thrift shops. Fashionable Honolulu men's stores began to stock real 'antique' shirts and when vintage shirts ran out, manufacturers 'dusted off history' and the recreations came off the line... Today (1979) there are 130 apparel manufacturers turning out "new" silkies, traditional mu`umu`u and aloha shirts.[76]

Several things converged to bring the silkies back into international consciousness. The simple designs of the sixties were considered boring, and in the haute couture salons of Europe nostalgia reigned supreme. Yves St. Laurent and Kenzo Okada brought out lines of clothing based on Tahitian prints. Fashion directors returned from the fashion showings in Europe ready for the new look. Dave Rochlen, from Surf Line Hawai`i noted that "their renaissance began in Europe. The Art Deco movement was important and this came together with a renewed willingness to revisit … the European concept of Polynesia as Paradise." At the same time, the quality of rayon had improved and polyester didn't sell as well due to its lack of breathability. Several designers put their reputations on the line brought out the 'new' silkies that looked surprisingly like the original silkies of the late 1940s and 1950s. Unfortunately, these designs were very slow to take hold in Hawai`i, and had to be sold on the mainland. The retro styles didn't catch on in Hawai`i until the eighties.[77]

Interest in Hawaiian quilting, a unique form of reverse appliqué, surged in the late 1970s. Mamo Howell is now well known for using Hawaiian quilt motifs on prints for aloha attire for both men and women. She began her business, (using the label 'Mamo'), in 1978 by producing lightweight summer quilts, then turned to the mu`umu`u. She felt the style needed an updating from the missionary look. Mamo initiated the 'demitasse' look that is somewhat shorter than full-length. "We revolutionized the mu`umu`u."[78]

From the 1930s to the 1970s, Consolidated Theatres had their usherettes wear white pleated pants, white shirts and leis. A uniform change occurred in the seventies when they required their usherettes to wear aloha shirts. Also in the 1970s, McDonalds (who came to Hawai`i in 1968) had their employees wear aloha shirts. Although minuscule at the time, identity apparel production would soon become a driving force in the Hawaiian garment industry.[79]

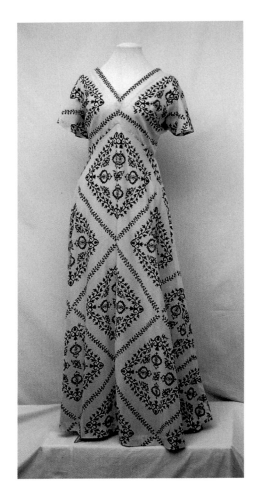

Cotton broadcloth mu`umu`u, *Mamo*,
1970s, 95.8.1, $100 to $299

Women's Attire

The casual dress of the mainland had an enormous impact
on aloha attire. The formality seen in the 1950s and 1960s was
gone, and with it the holomu`u and holoku became relegated
to use in only the most formal events, such as weddings and
Aloha Week (renamed Aloha Festivals in the 1980s). The
holoku was not fitted as closely as it had been in the previous
decade, and fuller skirts returned to holoku design. Traditional
holoku continued to be worn mostly by traditional and conservative women, such as members of the Ka'ahumanu Society who continued to dress in traditional black holoku. For
weddings in the 1970s, holoku design continued the trend of
reliance on turn of the century designs with high necklines
and leg-of-mutton sleeves.

The most important garment for women in the 1970s continued to be the mu`umu`u. Mini mu`umu`u, because they
were so short, were likely to be relatively simple and followed
design lines for apparel produced on the mainland. Often, the
only Hawaiian impact on the mini mu`u was its tropical or
floral fabrics. However, floral fabrics, in long flowing cotton
gowns were the vogue on the mainland in the 1970s, so consequently the same were seen in Hawaiian dress. Again, the use
of Hawaiian prints was the most noticeable feature of aloha
wear. Because the long mu`umu`u provided more room for
design, it was in these long dresses that the 1970s designers
felt free to include various design elements from other cultures. Traditional dress from Asia was a source of design inspiration, particularly from China and Japan. Some of the more
common ethnic details used in the 1970s included: asymmetri-
cal openings, accompanied by mandarin collars and fabric knot
buttons, reminiscent of Chinese dragon robes; kosode sleeves,
from Japanese kimono; the paneulo, a wide shawl-like collar
from the Philippines; and African inspired head wraps and
fabrics.

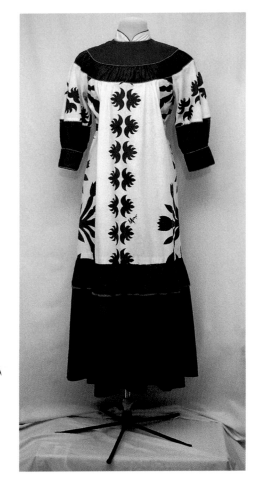

Cotton polyester blend mu`umu`u , *Mamo*, 1970s,
98.5.1, $100 to $299

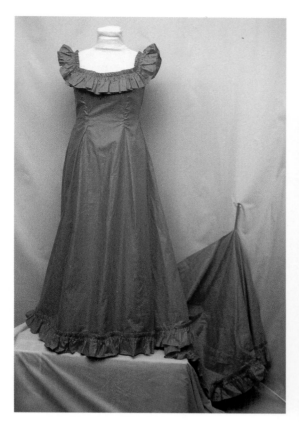

Cotton sateen holoku, custom made, 1970s, 96.1.1, $100 to $299

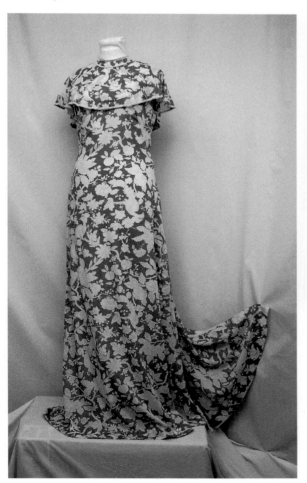

Cotton voile holoku, *Bete*, 1970s, 75.5.3, $100 to $299

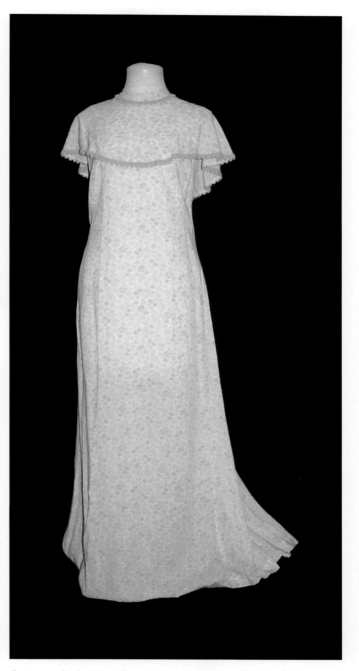

Cotton voile holoku, *Bete*, 1970s, TS96.11.1, $100 to $299

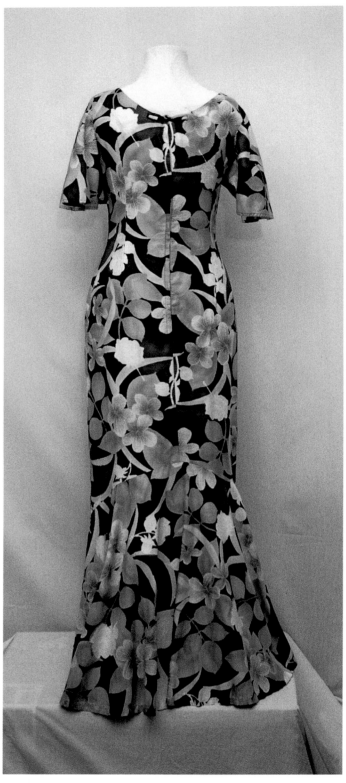

Cotton sateen holomu`u, *Kay's of Honolulu* , 1970s, 98.2.19,
$700 to $999

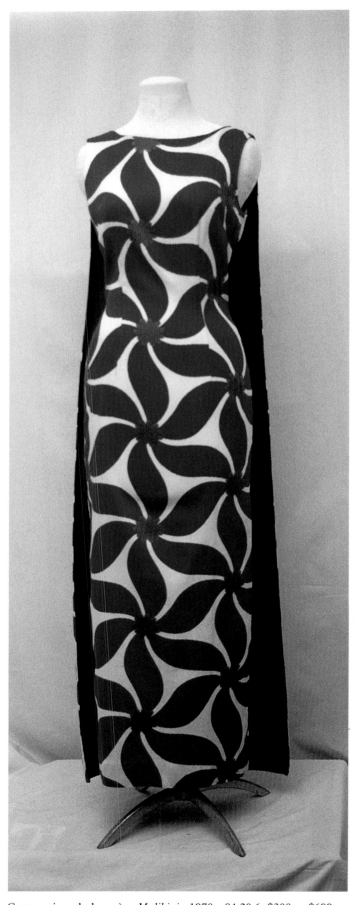

Cotton pique holomu`u, *Malihini* , 1970s, 84.20.6, $300 to $699

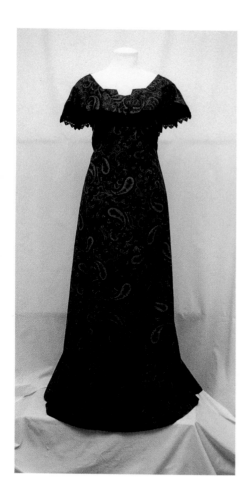

Cotton broadcloth mu`umu`u, "Luana" by *Bete, Courtesy of Bete, Inc.*, 1970s, $100 to $299

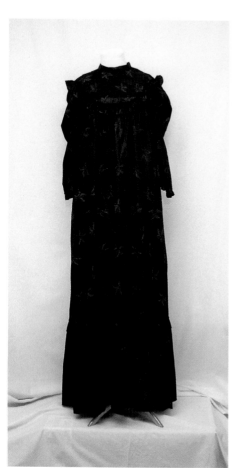

Cotton sateen mu`umu`u, *Andrade's Fine Resort Ap*parel, 1970s, 96.1.17, under $100

Mu`umu`u, $300 to $699, silk velvet with gold feather yoke, Custom made, *Courtesy of Barbara Harger*, 1970s, $300 to $699

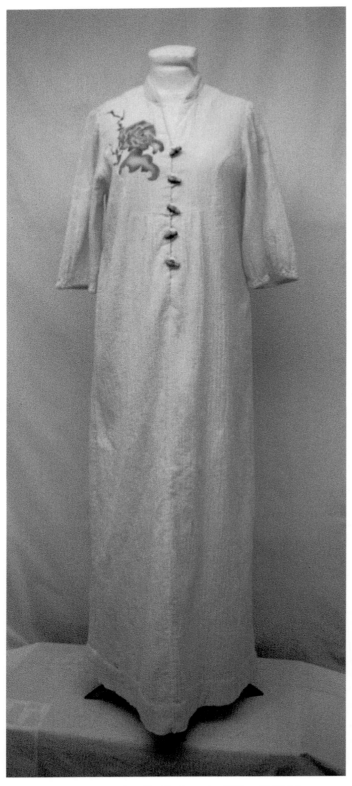

Cotton gauze mu`umu`u, *Dael's Casuals*, 1970s, 98.17.16,
$100 to $299

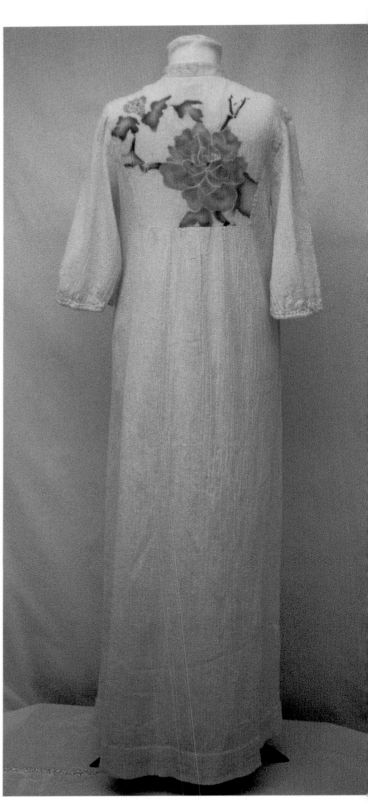

Cotton gauze mu`umu`u, (back) *Dael's Casuals*, 1970s, 98.17.16,
$100 to $299

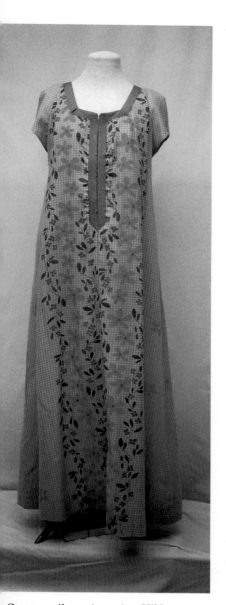

Cotton voile mu`umu`u, *Hilda Hawaii for Carol and Mary,* 1970s, 89.6.3, $100 to $299

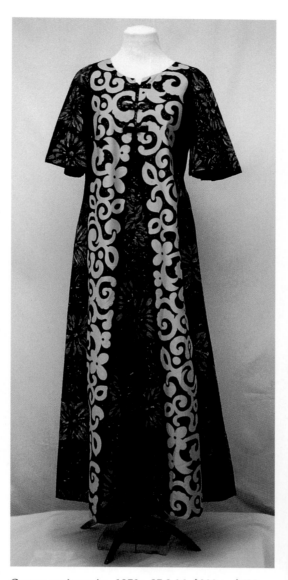

Cotton mu`umu`u, 1970s, 87.9.16, $300 to $699

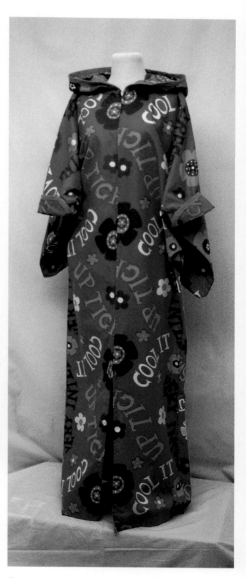

Cotton print mu`umu`u, with sayings from the TV show *Laugh In, Kamehameha,* 1970s, 86.8.82, $300 to $699

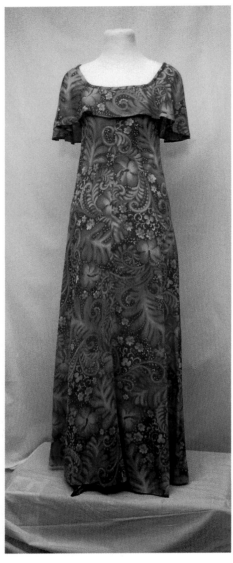

Acrylic mu`umu`u, 1970s 89.10.6, under $100

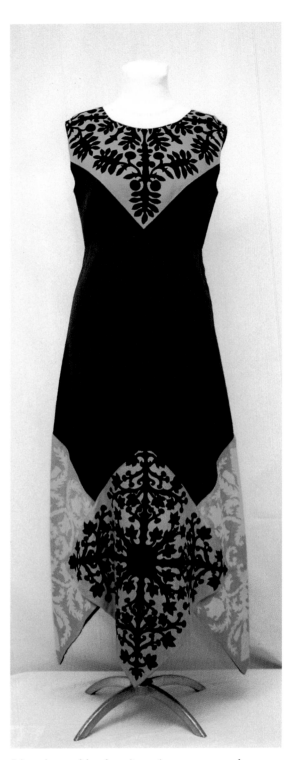

Linen/rayon blend mu`umu`u, custom made, Hawaiian quilt pattern in screen printed panels, 1970s, 79.14.2, $300 to $699

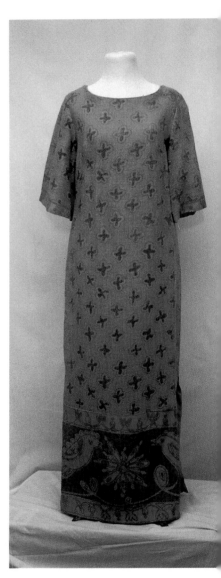

Cotton mu`umu`u, *Malihini*, 1970s 87.4.14, $100 to $299

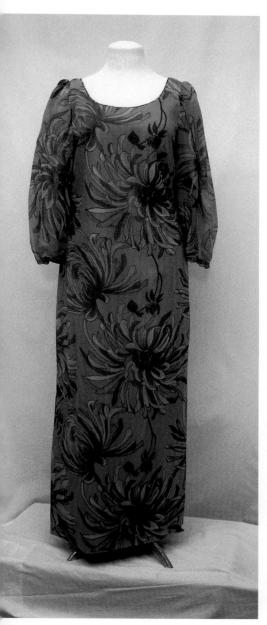

Nylon acetate mu`umu`u, *Kyomi for Liberty House,* 1970s, 87.4.2, $100 to $299

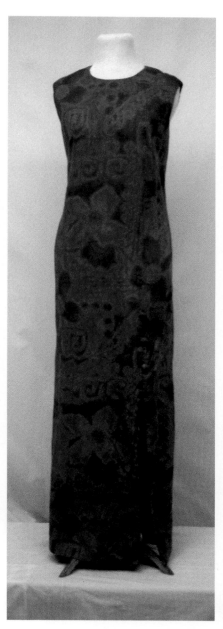

Polyester mu`umu`u, *Andrades,* 1970s, 76.29.47, $100 to $299

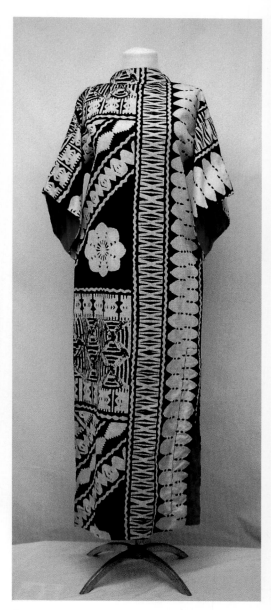

Cotton barkcloth mu`umu`u, *Guadalupe,* 1970s, 84.20.17, $100 to $299

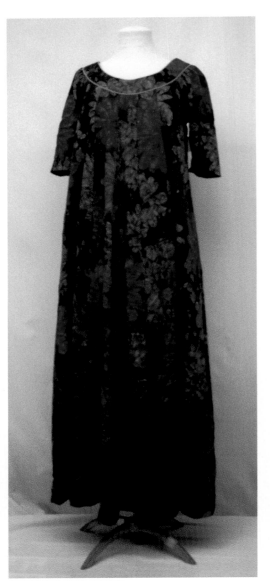

Acrylic mu`umu`u, Kyomi *for Liberty House,* 1970s, 96.1.33, $100 to $299

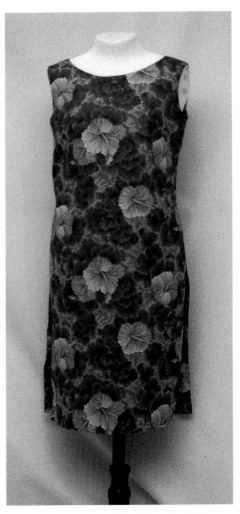

Acrylic mu`umu`u, *Kamehameha,* 1970s, 86.8.50, $100 to $299

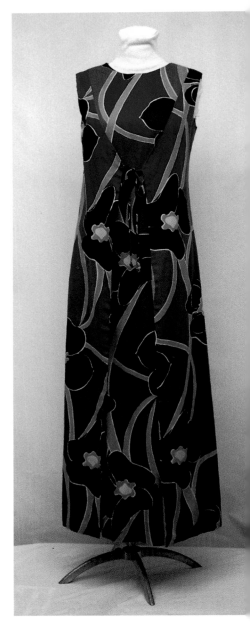

Cotton mu`umu`u, *Malihini,* 1970s, 84.20.20, $100 to $299

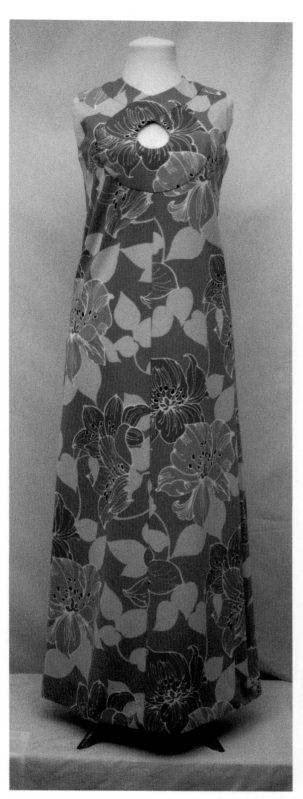

Polyester mu`umu`u, 1970s, 89.10.4, $100 to $299

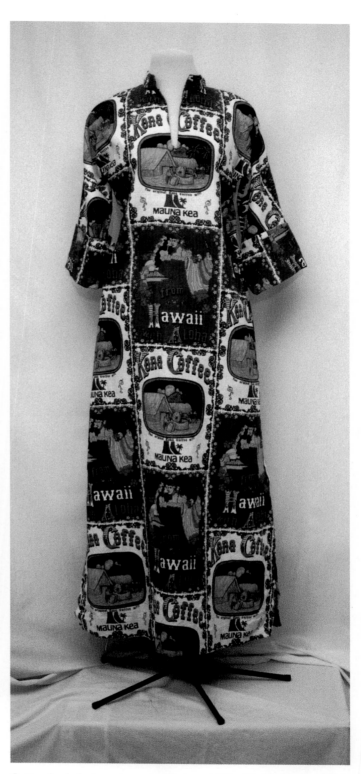

Cotton barkcloth mu`umu`u, *Esthers*, 1970s, 98.6.1, $100 to $299

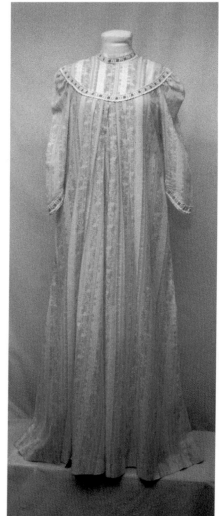

Cotton mu`umu`u, *Bete*, 1970s,
TS98.1.5, $100 to $299

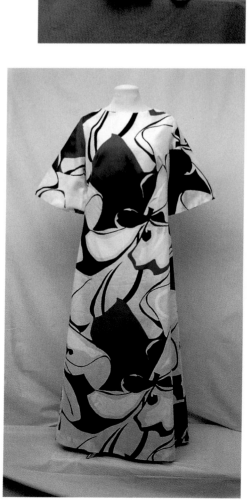

Cotton gingham mu`umu`u, custom made by Gloria Furer,
1970s, 94.7.1, $100 to $299

Cotton pique mu`umu`u, *Liberty House*,
1970s, 89.1.2, $100 to $299

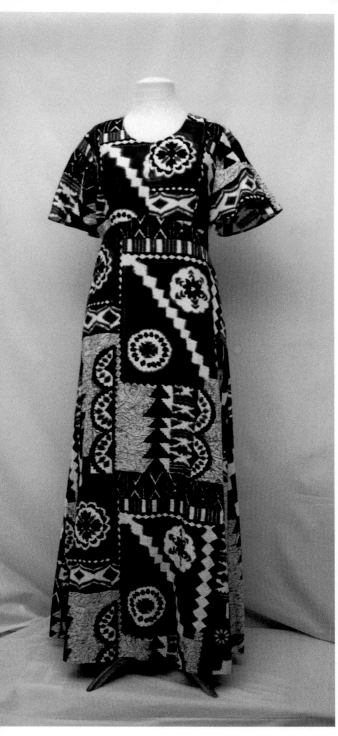

Cotton barkcloth mu`umu`u, 1970s, 87.9.4, $100 to $299

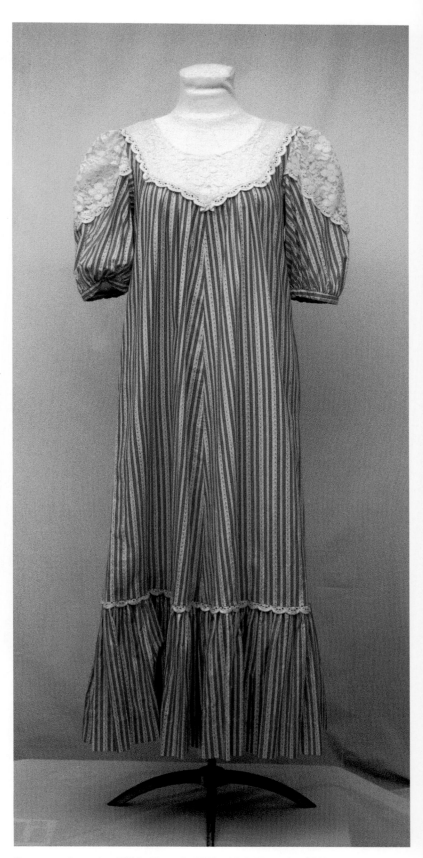

Cotton mu`umu`u, *Hilda Hawaii*, 1970s, 97.6.17, under $100

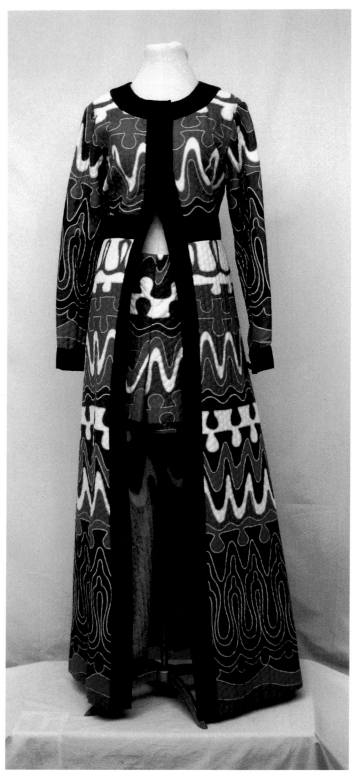

Mu`umu`u/hot pants in cotton waffle pique, *Tori Richard*,
1970s, 84.20.4, under $100

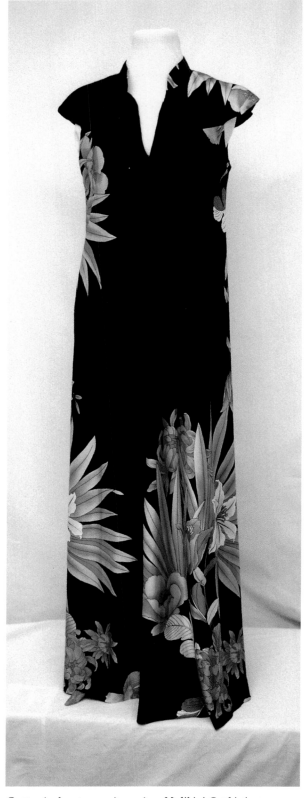

Cotton/polyester mu`umu`u, *Malihini Sophisticates*,
1970s, 95.10.5, under $100

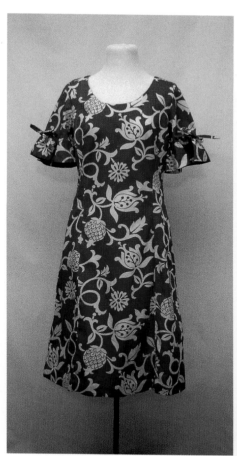

Cotton mu`umu`u, *Kamehameha*,
1970s, TS96.1.29, under $100

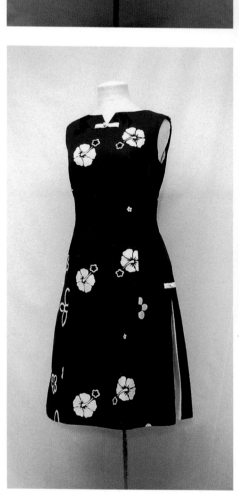

Cotton barkcloth mu`umu`u, 1970s, 99.1.111, under $100

Cotton mu`umu`u, *Kamehameha*,
1970s, 86.8.4, under $100

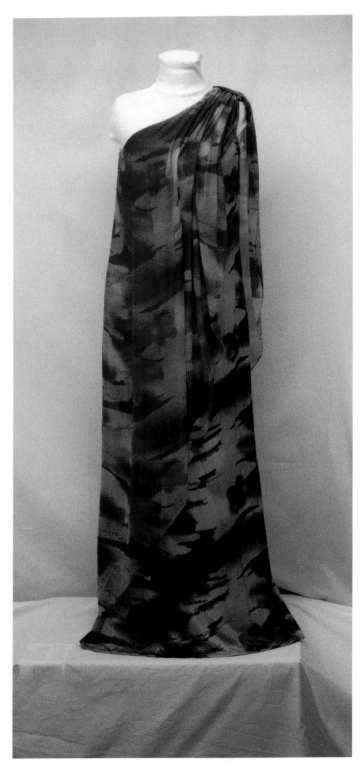

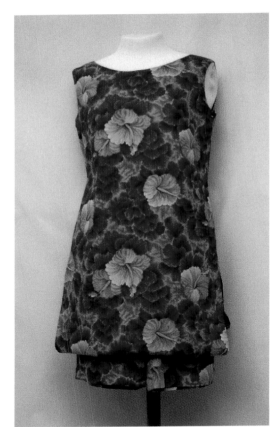

Cotton mu`umu`u and shorts, *Kamehameha*, 1970s, 86.8.50, $100 to $299

Nylon tricot mu`umu`u *Kamehameha* 1970s version of kihei, 86.8.35, under $100

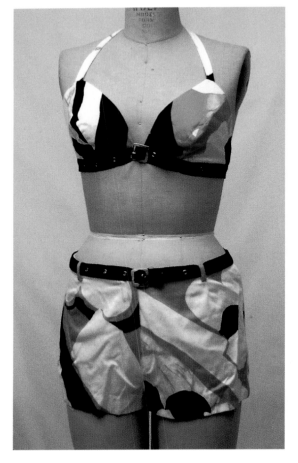

Swim bra with board shorts, cotton, *Kamehameha*, 1970s, 86.8.187, under $100

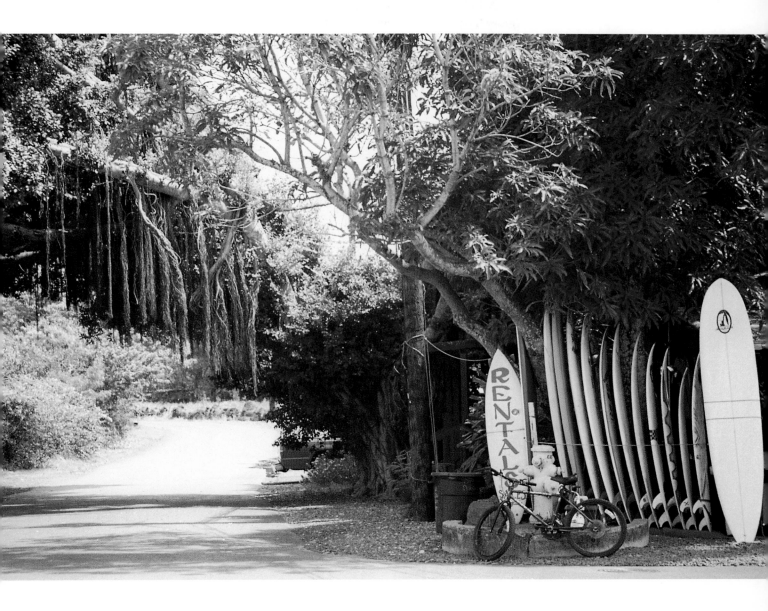

Men's Wear

The 1970s was a decade characterized by casual styles in the Western world. The 'Peacock Revolution' in menswear was a visual result of changing gender roles. The lines between masculine and feminine design details blurred. What had formerly been too feminine for a man's shirt, in terms of color, design, motifs and trims, became acceptable (at least for awhile) in American fashion. That had some impact on aloha shirts; they became rather wild in design during the 1970s. Hawaiian notions of gender were not as rigid as those on the mainland, and Hawaiian textile designs were less restrained as well. Although women had occasionally worn men's aloha shirts in Hawai`i for years, during the 1970s the aloha shirt became a unisex garment. "Men are accepting their feminine side. Males no longer have to be super macho in our society…Men and women feel comfortable in the same clothes. [Aloha shirts are] made to order for both sexes."[80]

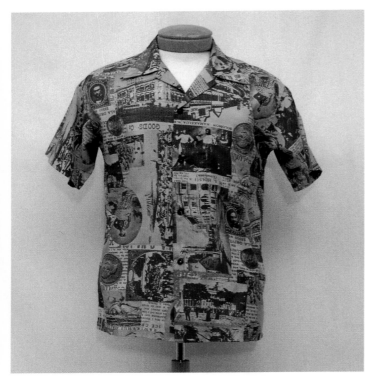

Nylon photo aloha shirt, *Himura*, 1973, *Courtesy of Kamehameha Garment Co.*, $300 to $699

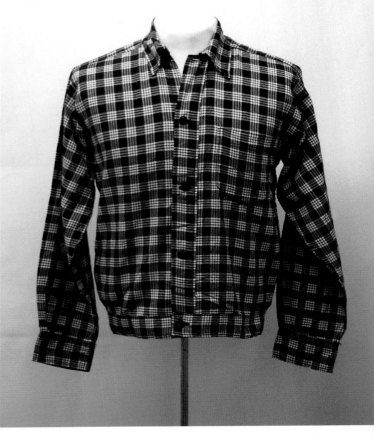

Palaka jacket, cotton, custom made in the 1970s of a pattern in constant use since the 1920s, *Courtesy of Barbara Kawakami*, 1970s, $300 *to* $699

In the late 1970s, when interest for the traditionally- styled aloha shirt was waning, Tori Richard and Kamehameha came out with new designs with softer shaping for men's shirts. Often, these were knit shirts that hugged the body; some were pullovers with slashed necklines and wild prints. To celebrate Tori Richard's twenty-fifth birthday and the opening of a new men's clothing department at Liberty House, Mort Feldman (President of Tori Richard) and the fine-jewelry department of Liberty House offered a $25,000 aloha shirt for sale. The long sleeved shirt was of silk, with bold leaf hand-screened design. With diamond and gold stays in the lapels and diamonds set in gold for the buttons, it was a most unique shirt.

By the late 1970s, there was a clear trend regarding aloha shirts; those worn by Hawaiian residents were usually more subdued than aloha shirts worn by tourists. The use of aloha shirts in the workplace became accepted practice, so long as the shirts had simple designs with regular repeats. The boldly patterned fabrics were considered a bit too shocking for the business world, and a compromise was made with reverse prints. Softer colors were used for business shirts, as opposed to casual aloha shirts. Since casual shirts in Hawai`i had generally been worn loose over the trousers, during the shift of aloha shirts into a business environment in the 1970s, there was much discussion as to the appropriate way to wear aloha shirts at the office. Eventually, the standard practice adopted was to wear the shirts tucked in. However, this has changed in recent years to less formality in Hawaiian offices, and the shirts can be worn either way, depending upon the nature and composition of the business.

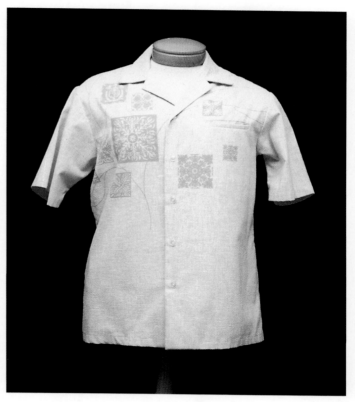

Cotton/polyester blend aloha shirt, *Iolani,* 1970s, 98.2.26, $100 to $299

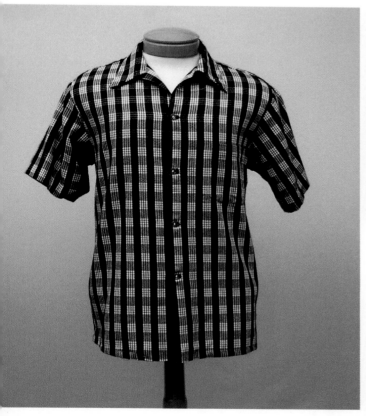

Palaka shirt, cotton/polyester, *Andrades,* 1970s, 98.5.1, $100 to $299

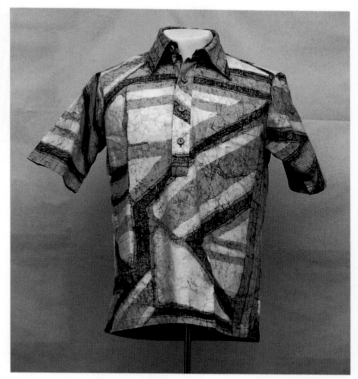

Cotton barkcloth aloha shirt, *Surfline,* 1970s, 94.4.1, $100 to $299

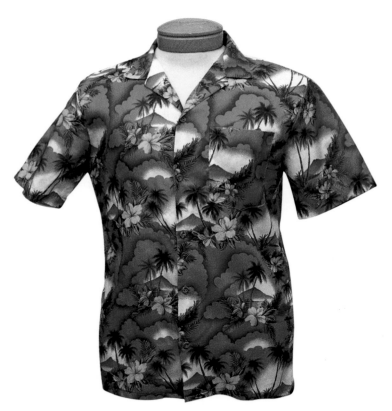

Polyester aloha shirt, *Islander*, 95.9.1, $100 to $299

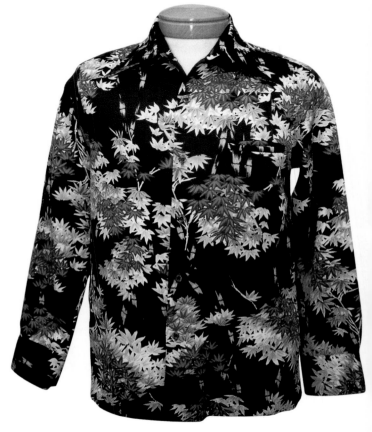

Polyester aloha shirt, *Tori Richard.* Long sleeve shirts were worn for dressy events. 1970s, 97.11.8, $100 to $299

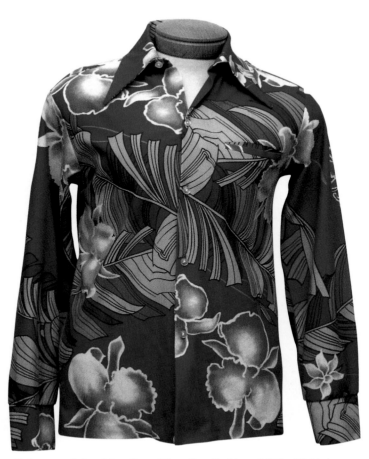

Polyester aloha shirt, *Sears Hawaiian Fashions*, 1970s, 94.11.4, $100 to $299

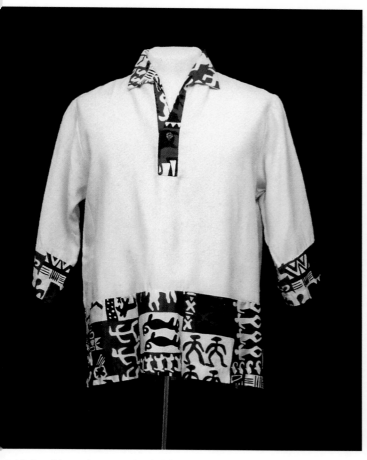

Aloha shirt, triacetate sharkskin with cotton border,
Kamehameha, 1970s, 86.8.144, $100 to $299

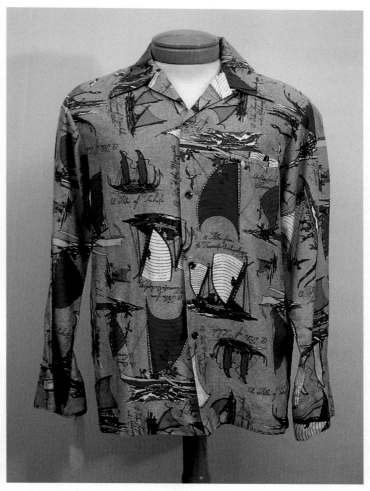

Cotton aloha shirt, *Sears Hawaiian Fashions,* , 1970s,
96.1.26, $100 to $299

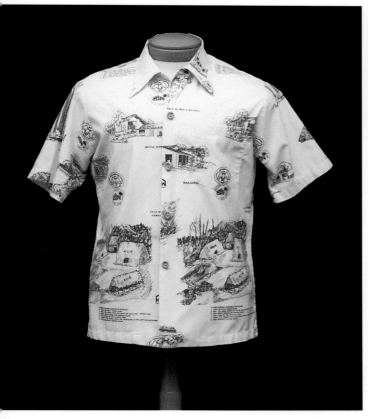

Rayon/cotton blend aloha shirt, *Action Sportswear,* 1970s, 94.11.1,
$100 to $299

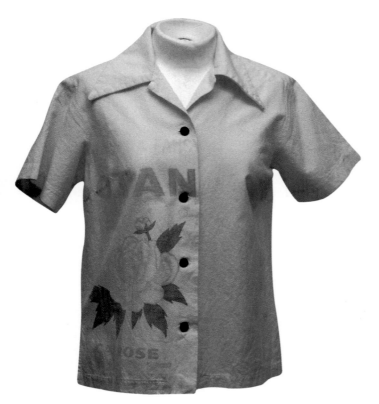

Woman's aloha shirt, cotton, custom made in the 1970s using rice bags in the 1940s style, 85.14.7, $100 to $299

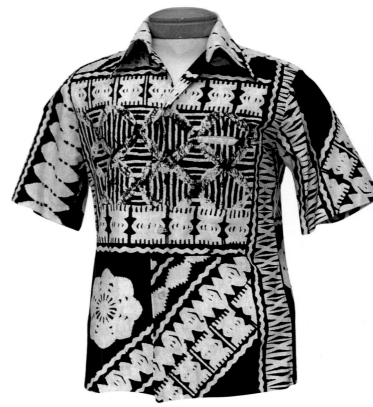

Cotton barkcloth aloha shirt, *Deone's Sportswear*, 1970s, 96.1.13, $100 to $299

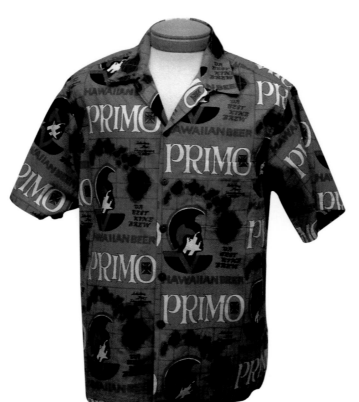

Cotton aloha shirt, *Go Barefoot*, 1970s, 98.2.25, $100 to $299

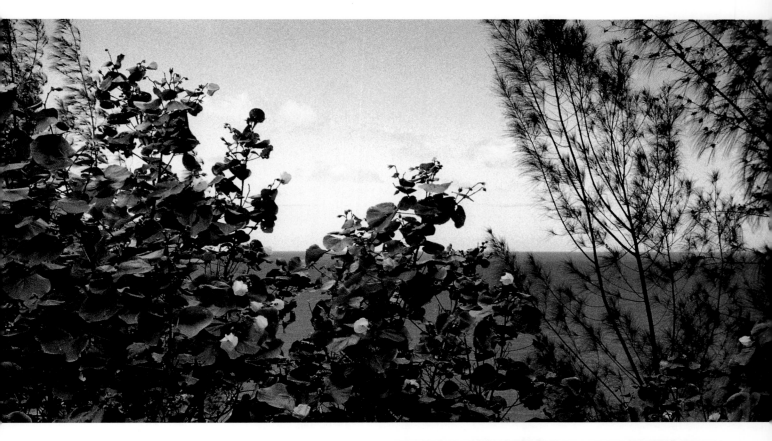

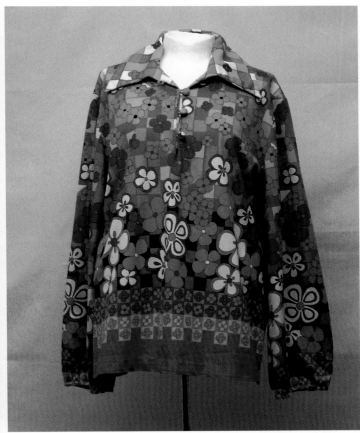

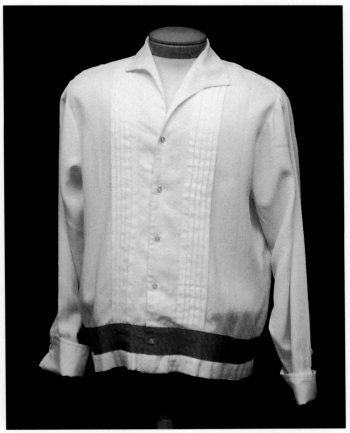

Polyester aloha shirt, *Napili*, 1970s, 86.6.3, $300 to $699

Triacetate aloha shirt, *Pua Pua Moa*, 1970s, 81.9.1, $100 to $299

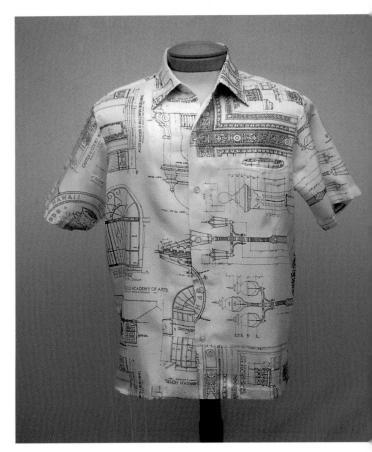

Polyester aloha shirt, *Tori Richard*, 1970s, 98.5.4, $100 to $299

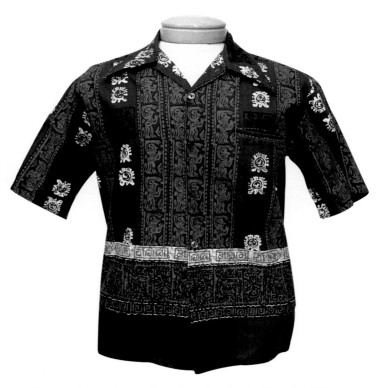

Cotton aloha shirt, batik design, *Barefoot in Hawaii*, 1972-1978,*Courtesy of Tony Gehringer*, 94.8.1, $100 to $299

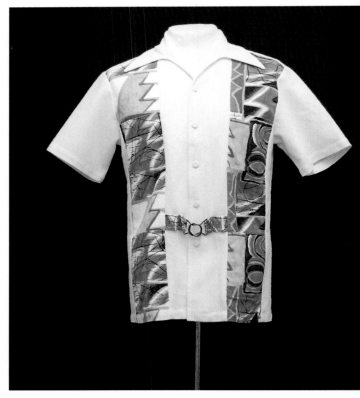

Cotton/polyester blend aloha shirt, *Iolani*, 1970s, TS96.1.16, under $100

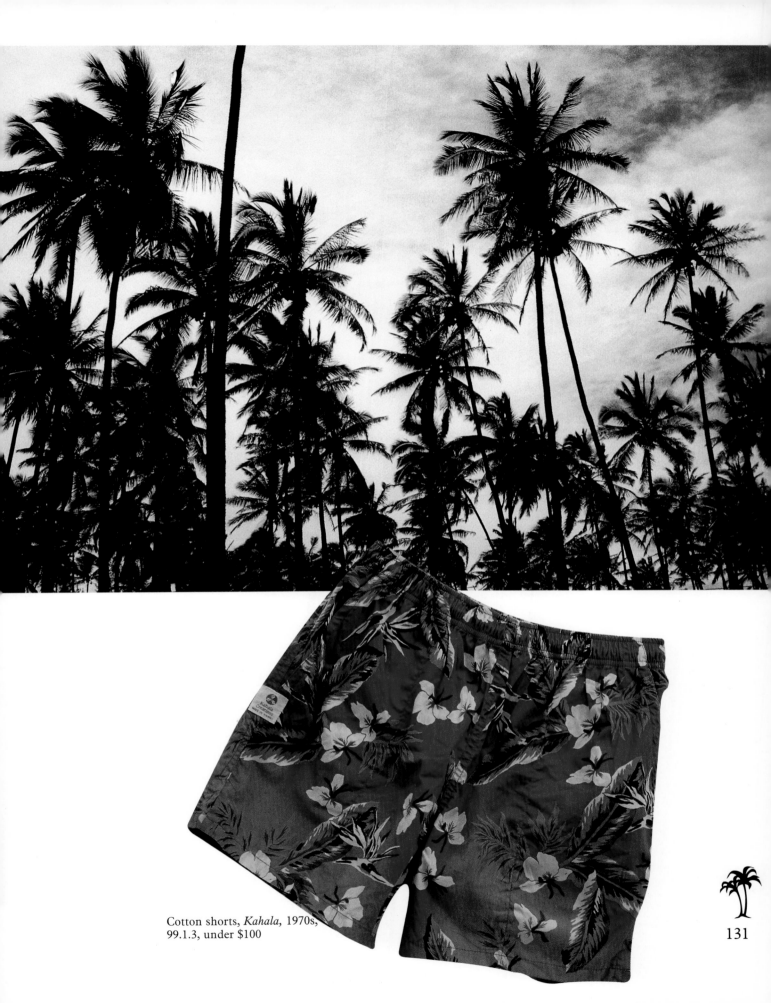

Cotton shorts, *Kahala*, 1970s,
99.1.3, under $100

9. The 1980s and 1990s
Hawaiian Renaissance & Retro Styles

Cultural Context

There is an enormous interest within Hawai`i regarding traditional Hawaiian culture and philosophy; this interest on the part of many locals in Hawai`i was re-awakened in the late 1970s and led to what has been termed 'The Hawaiian Renaissance.' The fundamental issue driving this interest was political, with continuing unrest in the State of Hawai`i, most especially by native Hawaiians, over the unjust overthrow of the Hawaiian monarchy in 1893. Some history is pertinent here. The Kingdom of Hawai`i was recognized internationally as a sovereign country. It had valid treaties with many nations, including the United States. In 1893, a group of (predominantly white) American businessmen, backed by U.S. Marines, illegally overthrew the Hawaiian monarchy and took control. Although President Cleveland condemned the act and called for the restoration of the Hawaiian monarchy, in violation of both US and international law, President McKinley pushed through a resolution of annexation in 1898. In 1900 Hawai`i was a territory of the US, then a state in 1959, but today many people challenge the legitimacy of this vote and of statehood itself. "In 1993, the U.S. Congress and President Clinton officially apologized for the overthrow, acknowledging the illegality of it and the annexation, and recognizing the inherent sovereignty and right to self-determination of Native Hawaiians. Today the Hawaiian sovereignty movement is highly active, and even mainstream political leaders recognize that it is not a matter of if, but when and in what form sovereignty will come to the islands."[81]

The Hawaiian sovereignty movement parallels the cultural renaissance which began to gather steam in the late 1970s after the Hokule`a made its first voyage. This stimulated a renaissance of Hawaiian arts and crafts, as well as the performing arts. "It became important in the late 1970s with the performing and visual arts." Valerie Taylor, head designer for Dano, remembered going to watch Hawaiian musicians Keola and Kapono Beamer at the Territorial Tavern and wondered how she could capture that Hawaiian spirit in her designs. "We were there almost every night. Trying to put our minds into the old Hawaiian style. I started looking for something to wear to the tavern and bought some original men's silkies at $150 each. I tied the ends at the waist and everyone liked them. After awhile it just seemed natural to be thinking in terms of recreating the old silkies."[82]

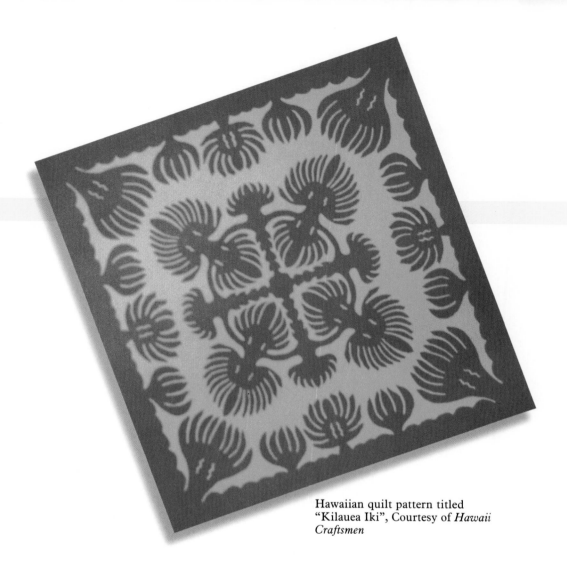

Hawaiian quilt pattern titled "Kilauea Iki", Courtesy of *Hawaii Craftsmen*

Fabrics

With a fine arts background, Alan James is one of several textile artists seeking to replace the "hash" prints of yesteryear with culturally meaningful textiles. His fabrics are often subtle two-color designs featuring a particular item of importance to Hawaiian culture. For example, lei are given to represent a person's accomplishments, and the 'ilima lei indicates pride and achievement. These colorful lei are featured in one of his designs. Similarly, the kukui nut is symbolic as well, historically considered to be indicative of knowledge. Other designs feature canoes, quilts, and Hawaiian flora. The kahili and crown of the Hawaiian monarchy are found in some of his artwork as well. Several other artists also intentionally use Hawaiian motifs in order to embed cultural values into fabric.

Ideas for Tori Richard's lifestyle prints come from their extensive archives, developed over the past half-century. Tori Richard has 3,000-4,000 archival prints collected from books, magazines, fine art of all kinds, trends and trips to European fashion capitals. A screen from India became the inspiration for a Tori Richard print called 'Tiger Hunt.' The Las Vegas-Hawai`i connection inspired neon brights on black with cowgirls, a deck of cards, motel signs, cactus and a jukebox. A book of concept cars that Detroit never built became 'Futurama

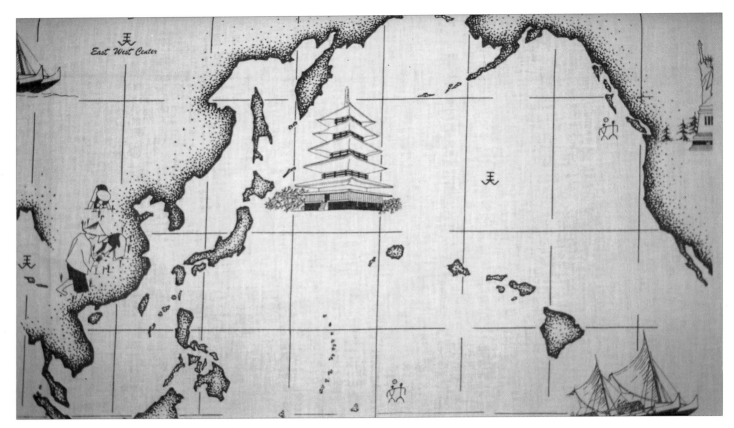

Linen map print for Hawaii's East-West Center

Cars.' Similarly, at Kahala Sportswear, much of the textile design comes from fine artists who apply their vision to fabric. Maui's Avi Kiriaty has created more than 200 prints for Kahala.

> My inspiration comes from the ocean and simply from living in paradise' says Kiriaty. … 'the ocean is all around us and is important to our survival, he says 'so it should always be in the forefront of our thoughts and our clothing. We must remember the ocean is a resource to be managed appropriately; there's a subtle environmental message in my work.

Chairman Dave Rochlen of Jams World® (a company that is known for its ebullient use of color in gregarious prints) says, "We're inspired by our credo: color, freedom, difference, love. We are artists reproducing life in all its joyous moods and we will create whatever provokes joy in living."[83]

Clothing Production

The demand for Hawaiian clothing on the mainland diminished in the late 1970s and early 1980s. Shaheen retained his factory and retail stores on the Islands during that time, but moved his design department to Los Angeles. Consequently, Shaheen began a gradual move away from the Hawaiian market and into the mainland market. However, the demand for Hawaiian music, food and aloha shirts on the mainland - especially in the western states - is increasing as the century comes to an end. Numerous mainland companies sell Hawaiian shirts over the internet, and one Hawaiian company, Hilo Hattie, has recently opened a store in Southern California.[84] Tori Richards and Kamehameha also do a great deal of business on the US mainland and Japan.

134

Apparel production is a very cyclical business, and aloha attire is even more prone to ups and downs than other forms of garment production. It is periodically the rage on the mainland, often due to the influence of celebrities from movies and television. Since the 1950s, the aloha shirt has been brought into mainstream consciousness by Arthur Godfrey, Harry Truman, Elvis Presley, Bing Crosby and in the 1980s, Tom Selleck (Magnum PI). International haute couture took notice, and began to produce tropical prints for mens wear and womens wear in the 1980s. Hanae Mori, Karl Lagerfeld and other top designers featured island themes in their lines, as they counteracted the heavy menswear influence of the early 1980s as comfortable and casual lifestyles gained favor. "No longer are Hawaiian fashions considered a novelty you stick in the back of the closet when you get back home."[85]

The Hawaiian garment industry represents the largest group of manufacturers in Hawai`i today (1999) and represents sales of one-half billion dollars annually. Apparel manufacturers export 30 percent of their products to the mainland US and other countries; $165 million dollars worth of apparel is exported internationally on an annual basis. Much of the renewed interest in aloha apparel has to do with the global appeal of it's recent shift toward resort apparel that features Hawaiian prints with more career-oriented garment lines.[86]

Alan James is one of the apparel manufacturers who is producing resort apparel with a more cosmopolitan appearance. James got into the aloha attire market in 1986. He produces aloha attire and identity apparel, including upscale blazers and professional clothing for women. He designs with the intention of recapturing Hawaiian culture in his textiles. Similarly, Puamana Crabbe, a 1981 graduate in fashion design from the University of Hawai`i at Manoa, designs with a focus on Hawaiian tradition. Designs by Puamana Crabbe began with garments for hula dancers and groups. Her aloha attire features appliquéd quilt patterns directly appliquéd onto the garments. Like Mamo, she also has some of her fabric silk-screened with quilt motifs.

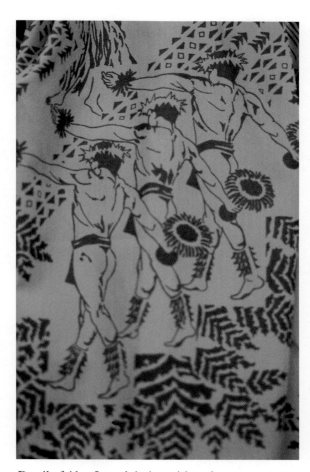

Detail of Alan James' design with male hula dancers, *Courtesy of Alan James*

By 1988 at least 150 garment manufacturers were in Hawai`i and they generated $120 million in sales. Three big changes in retail had an impact on the aloha attire industry: 1) local department stores began acquiring aloha attire offshore, so local manufacturers could not compete on price, 2) the introduction of "Big Box" retailers, like Wal-Mart, Kmart, and Costco, and 3) the beginning of swap meets in the 1970s at the Aloha Stadium and Kam Drive-In. These swap meets sold new garments, fabric and other Hawaiian goods. The Mu`umu`u Factory to You, which grew to nine locations by 1987 and sold mu`umu`u for under $26, was hard for the major manufacturers to compete with at prices of $50 to $60. "That made a big impact on the market," said Carol Zawtocki, current owner of Malihini. Three to four thousand people lost jobs as local apparel manufacturers reeled over the last decade. One company president said, "What really killed us was the swap meet," it enabled sewers to buy fabric and sell to the public at wholesale prices.[87]

As a result of the consumer's shift toward less expensive retail outlets, aloha attire manufacturers had to find other customers. The most significant shift in aloha attire production has been from the garment industry's prior focus that catered to tourists to making identity apparel. Several of the Hawaiian producers now produce aloha attire uniforms for workers in the tourism industry. Malihini Sportswear Inc., saw its aloha apparel manufacturing business shrink from five million dollars a year at the end of the 1970s to a half-million twenty years later, switched to uniform production to sustain the business. Malia Hawai`i Inc. from the 1960s is today, Uniforms By Malia. This company made sports and boutique wear for retail stores in Hawai`i and around the world in the 1960s and 1970s, but now is primarily manufacturing uniforms with an annual revenue of nearly one million dollars. Similarly, Tori Richard Ltd., began making uniforms in 1973 but recently found that their uniform division provides about a quarter of its sales. Tori Richard relied more on a renewed focus on the mainland to reinvigorate the company, which has seen double-digit sales growth in the last three years. Retail, however, remains tough. "It's a very tough industry," said the Mamo Howell, who does about forty percent of her business in identity apparel.[88]

Woman's Attire

Since the 1980s, the holoku has consistently reflected Hawaii's past rather than contemporary western or Hawaiian fashion. Design details from the turn of the century, such as white fabrics, from simple cottons to lace, are commonly found in contemporary holomu`u and holoku. During the 1980s, people in Hawai`i became more retrospective as the state prepared for the centennial anniversary of the overthrow of the Hawaiian monarchy. Focus on Hawaiian culture led to a resurgence of turn-of-the-century designs for both holomu`u and holoku. Long sleeves and ruffles returned in the 1980s and continue today. Turn of the century styles, with pin tucks, ruffles, high necklines and leg-o-mutton sleeves have become favorites for both brides and flower girls.

Members of the Kaahumanu Society continue to honor the greatest Hawaiian female of them all, the favorite wife of Kamehameha, ... who led Hawaii's first women's liberation movement [in 1819] which overthrew the kapus that denied females...the eating of choice foods... Later, she held the reigns of government in her capable hands with a will of iron. The ladies of the Kaahumanu Society wear black in her memory. ... They still wear somber black, broken only by vivid yellow leis. Black dresses [holoku and mu`umu`u]. Black shoes. Black gloves. Black hats. To note the presence of the Kaahumanu Society at a social occasion is to know that it is one of historical Hawaiian significance.[89]

136

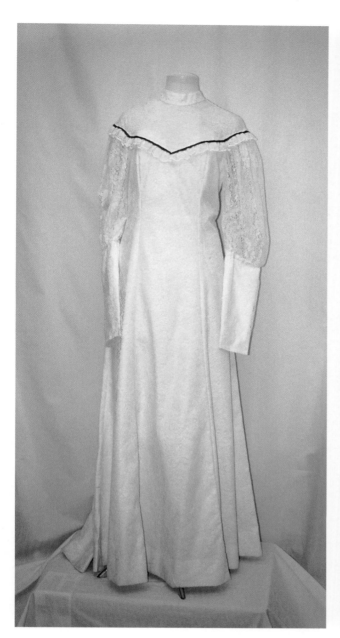

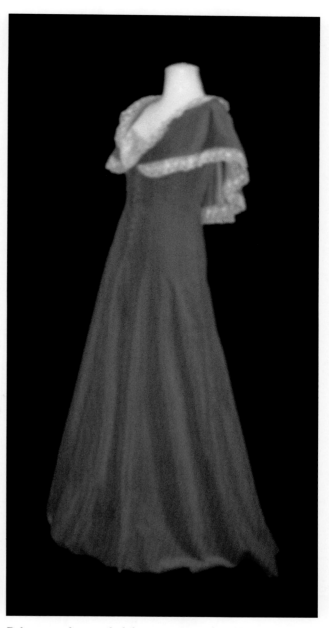

Lace holoku, *Popouai-Honolulu*, 1980s, 97.6.25, $300 to $699   Polyester velveteen holoku, custom made, 1980s, 95.4.1, $100 to $299

Traditional aloha attire has become a preferred form of dress for certain events, particularly rites of passage such as the baby luau, graduations and weddings. The holoku is worn for weddings, the holoku Ball and Aloha Festivals. Dress codes requesting aloha attire will be made clear on invitations to parties, and even in funeral announcements. "Hawai`i is evolving one of the most complicated dress codes in the nation," according to Bob Krauss, a reporter for the Honolulu Advertiser. When he arrived in Honolulu several decades ago, the newspaper had a dress code requiring reporters to wear coats and ties. Women wore gloves for shopping downtown, and the society editor wore hats to the office. The style was definitely formal. Krauss observed the evolution of Honolulu's dress codes, and noted that while lobbying by the garment industry pushed aloha wear as appropriate for business dress, some manufacturers made a great deal more profit on selling suits and tried to halt the slide into casual dress, without success. Although mu`umu`u and holomu`u are worn by many women, female executives rarely don aloha attire in public. The president of a public relations firm invited a large group of executive women to a tea, and none arrived in a mu`umu`u. Western dress or suits, and always with pantyhose, are the rule for executive women.[90]

Aloha attire for women has been evolving since the 1980s due to changes in women's social and professional roles. Women began to work outside the home in greater numbers, the Hawaiian lifestyle became more casual and dress became more comfortable. Along with social changes came a shift in dress considered appropriate for work

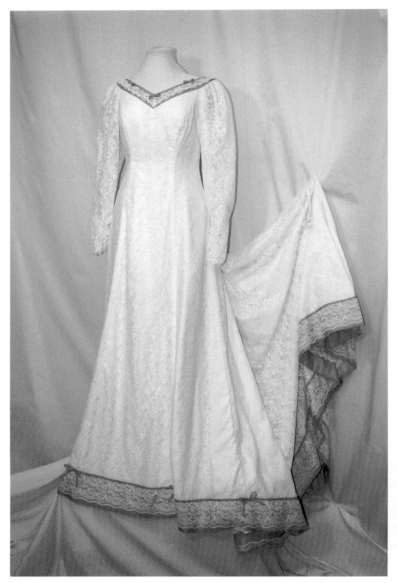

Lace and taffeta holoku, white, custom made, 1980s, 95.5.1, $300 to $699

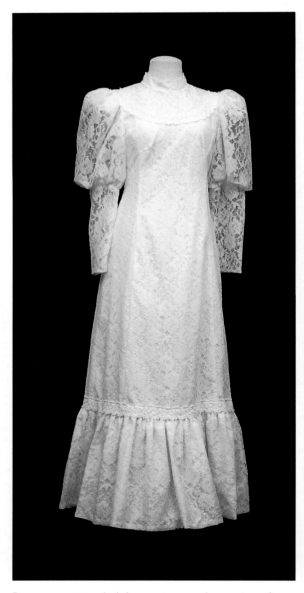

Lace over cotton holoku, custom made, *courtesy of Marla Nakata*, 1980s, $300 to $699

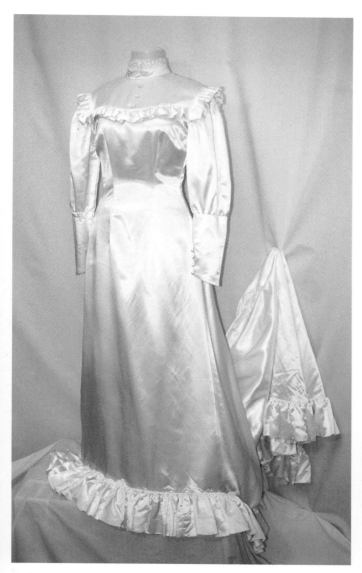

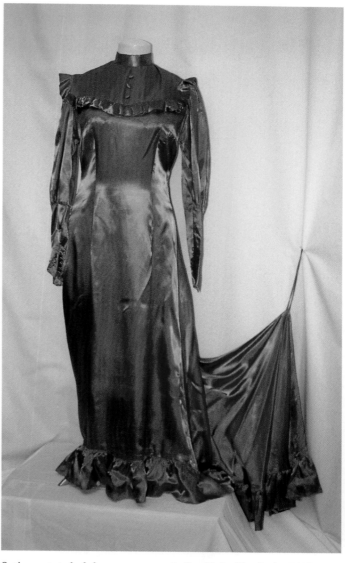

Satin acetate holoku, custom made for Aloha Festivals, 1980s, 97.9.1, $300 to $699

Satin acetate holoku, custom made for Aloha Festivals, 1980s, 98.2.15, $300 to $699

and for the "on the move" lifestyle of the 1980s. Comfort became critical for women's clothing and traditional aloha apparel had to change. The holomu`u has loosened somewhat and is now commonly referred to as a "tea length" mu`umu`u. (Early versions of the holomu`u could be cumbersome to walk in due to deep ruffles between the knee and hem). A clear shift in styling is occurring in the women's wear of the 1990s with a change from traditional aloha attire toward contemporary resort wear. Although Hawaiian prints are the focus of the contemporary aloha attire, it features a more cosmopolitan look in terms of simple, sleek design lines. While these garments may be body conscious, in that they often fit the body closely, they do not rely on ruffles and frills to assert femininity. The look is more tailored and generally more appropriate for career dress. Hotels have found this career look to be well suited toward pairing a Hawaiian sense of place with professional dress. For example, one hotel has their female employees wear Hawaiian print sarong skirts, tank tops and jackets.[91]

139

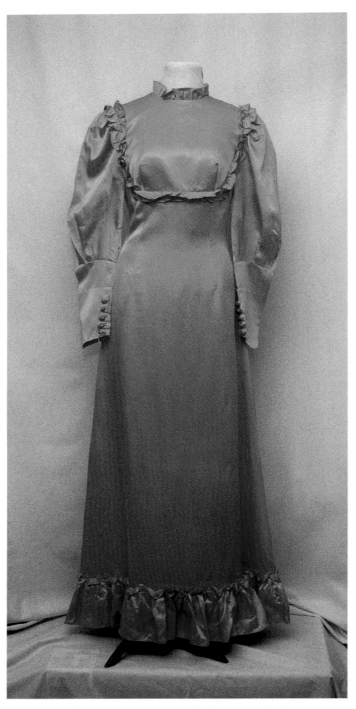

Satin acetate holomu`u, custom made for Aloha Festivals,
1980s, 97.9.2, $100 to $299

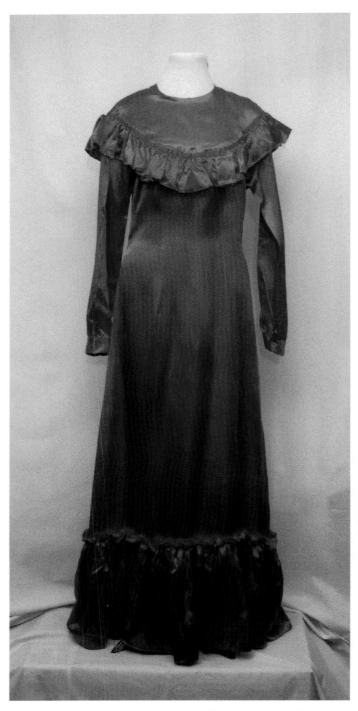

Satin acetate holomu`u, custom made for Aloha Festivals,
1980s, 98.2.20, $100 to $299

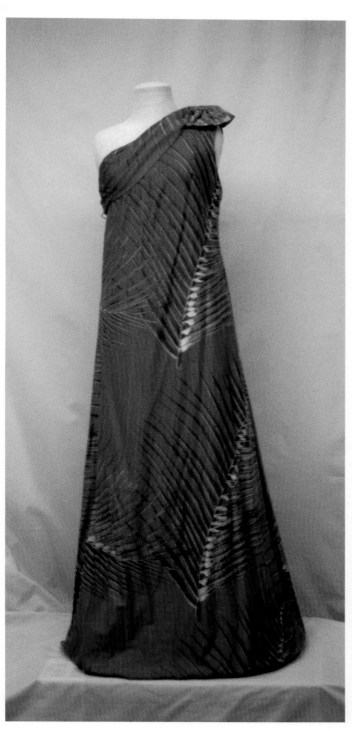

Cotton mu`umu`u, 80's version of the kihei, *Cecilia Sonza*,
84.22.150, under $100

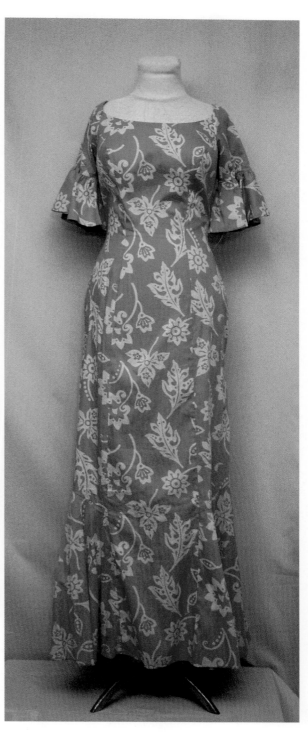

Cotton holomu`u, *Kamehameha*, 1980s, 86.8.156,
$100 to $299

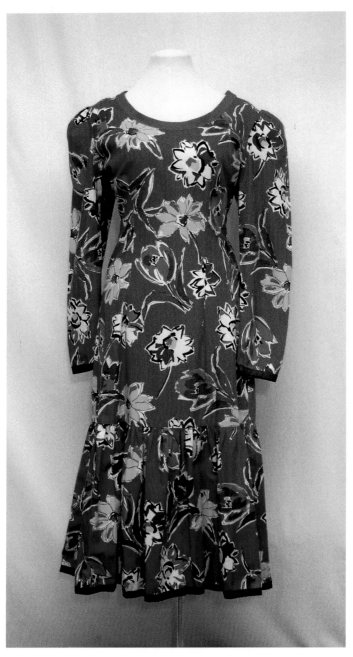

Cotton holomu`u, *Deborah Boutique*, 1980s, 96.1.2, $100 to $299

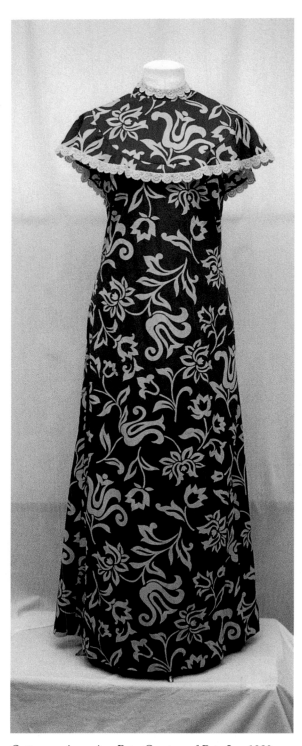

Cotton mu`umu`u, *Bete, Courtesy of Bete Inc.* 1980s, $100 to $299

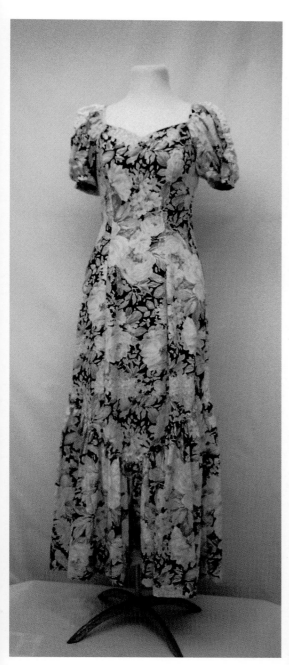

Cotton holomu`u, *Lola Jrs,* 1980s, 98.17.5,
$100 to $299

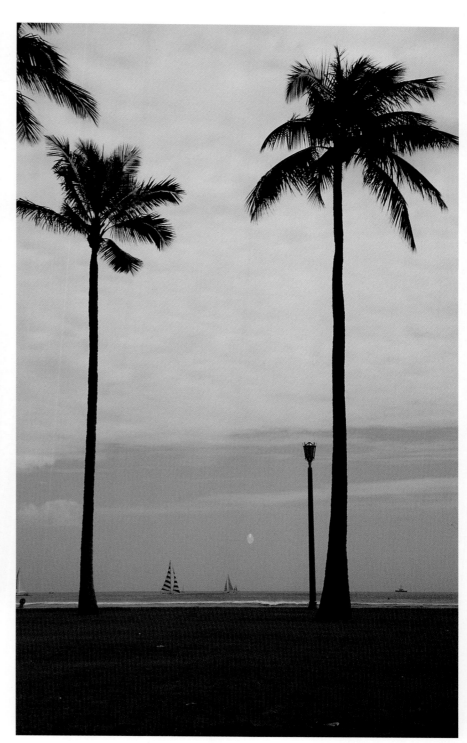

143

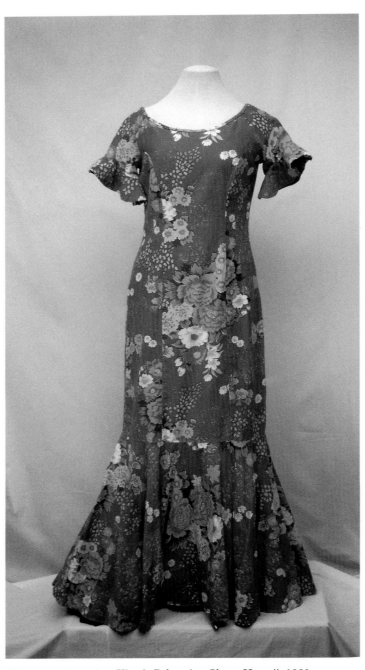

Cotton mu`umu`u, *Kimo's Polynesian Shore, Hawaii*, 1980s,
97.6.15, $100 to $299

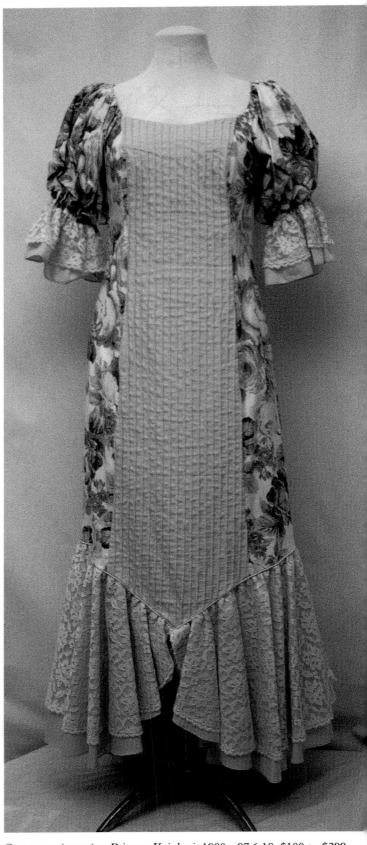

Cotton mu`umu`u, *Princess Kaiulani*, 1980s, 97.6.18, $100 to $299

144

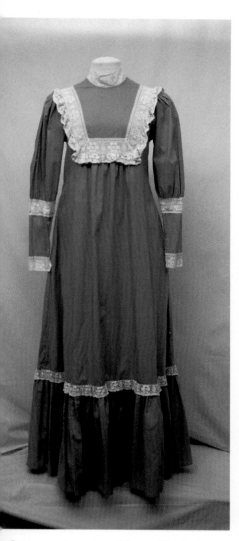

Cotton mu`umu`u, *Princess Kaiulani*,
1980s, 98.2.16, under $100

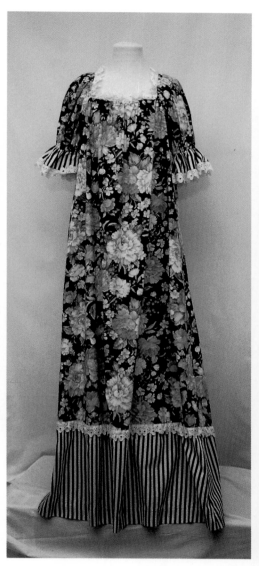

Cotton mu`umu`u, *Princess Kaiulani*, 1980s,
96.1.35, under $100

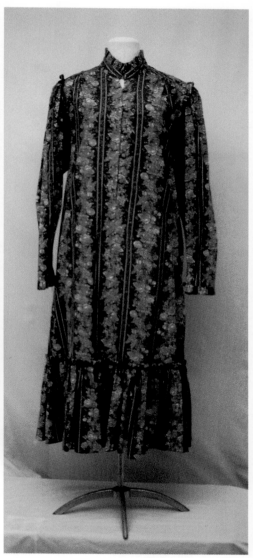

Cotton mu`umu`u, *Princess Kaiulani*,
1980s, 97.6.22, under $100

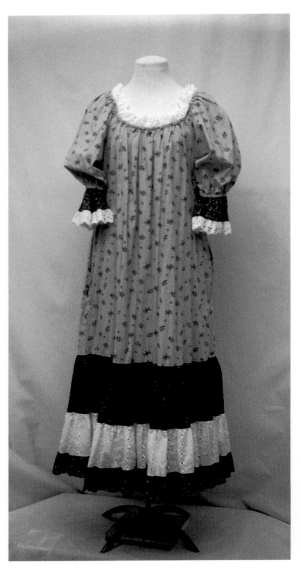

Cotton mu`umu`u, *Princess Kaiulani,* 1980s,
97.6.20, under $100

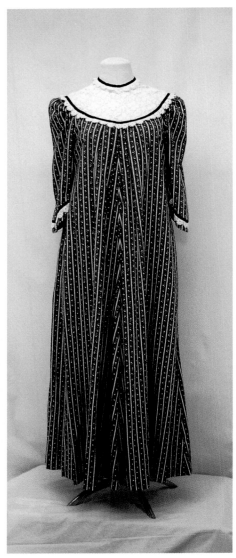

Cotton mu`umu`u, *Bete Collection,*
Andrade Shops, 1980s, 97.6.21, under $100

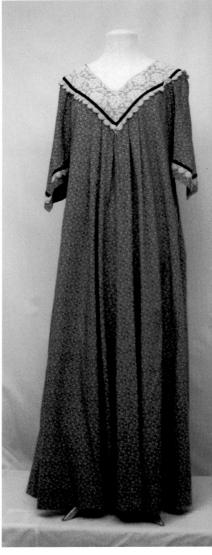

Cotton mu`umu`u, *Bete*
Collection, Andrade Shops, 1980s,
95.3.2, under $100

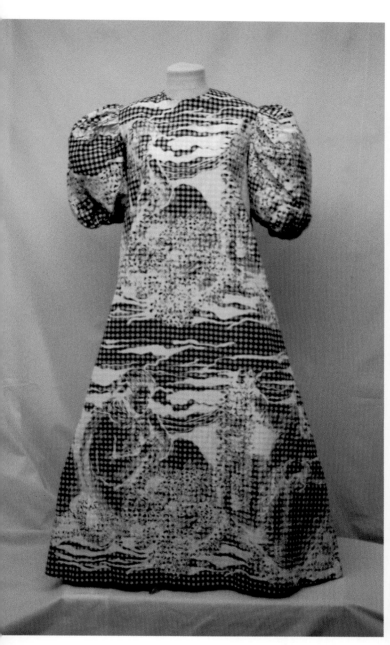

Cotton mu`umu`u designed by *Alan Akina*: the design is of a
woman making lei (screen printed over navy gingham), 1980s,
94.9.1, $100 to $299

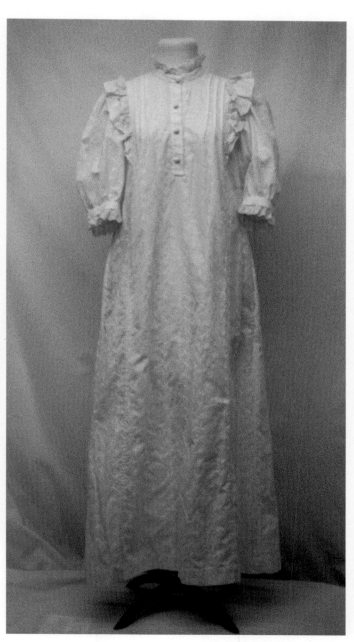

Cotton eyelet mu`umu`u, *Fumi's Originals*, 1980s, 98.2.17,
under $100

147

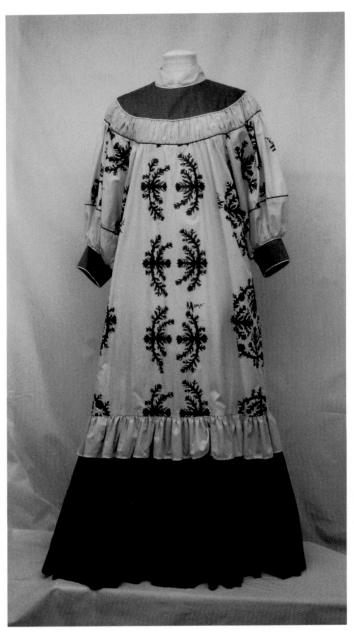

Cotton blend mu`umu`u, *Mamo*: (design of Hawaiian quilt motifs)1980s, 96.6.2, $100 to $299

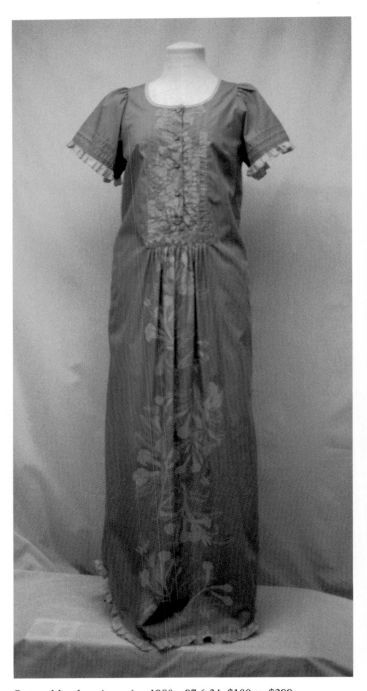

Cotton blend mu`umu`u, 1980s, 97.6.24, $100 to $299

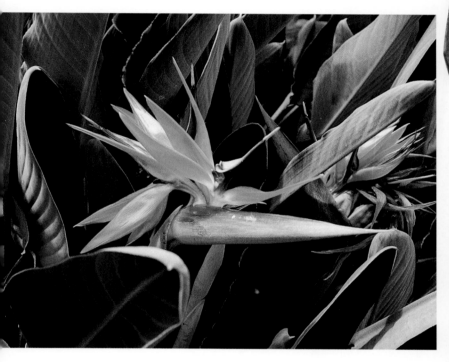

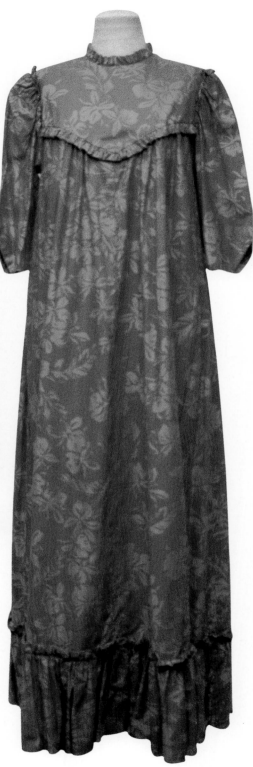

Cotton blend mu`umu`u, 80s version of 50s pareau print, *Mildred's of Hawaii* 89.4.2, under $100

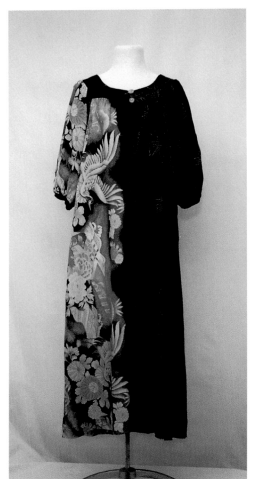

Rayon mu`umu`u, *Chix*,
96.1.30, $100 to $299

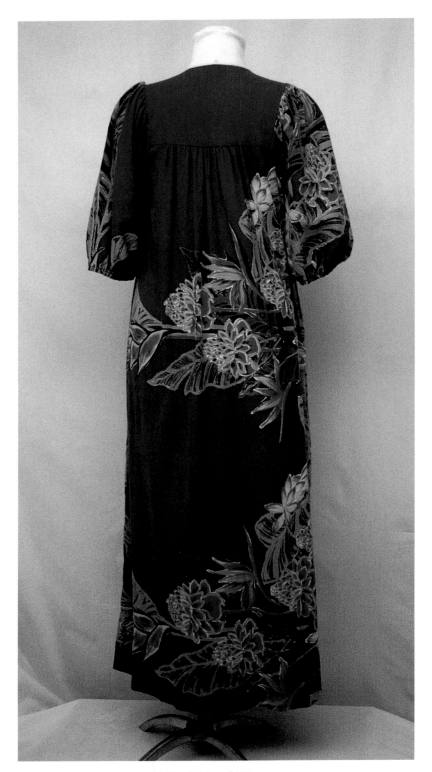

Rayon gauze mu`umu`u, 1980s, $100 to $299

150

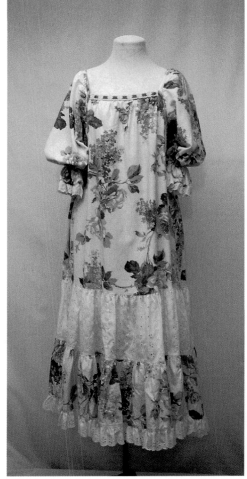

Cotton eyelet mu`umu`u, *Sears*,
1980s, 96.2.1, $100 to $299

Rayon mu`umu`u, *Cooke Street (Tori Richard)*, 1980s, 96.4.5, under $100

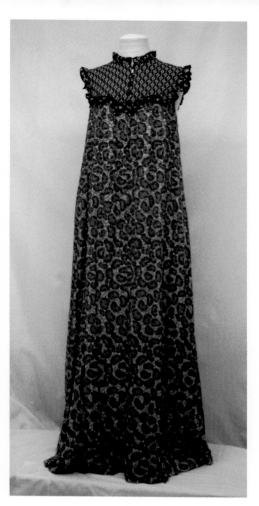

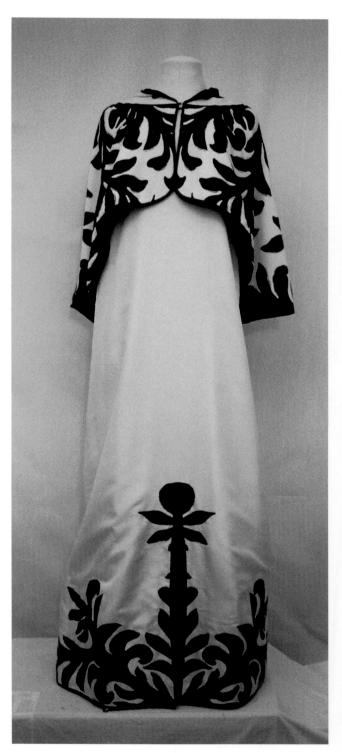

Silk blend mu`umu`u and cape, custom made with appliquéd Hawaiian quilt motif, 83.17.1, $300 to $699

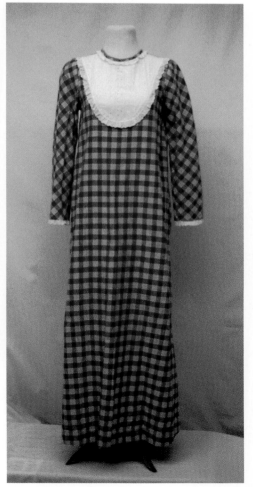

Cotton palaka mu`umu`u, *Potpourri Patch*, 1980s, 96.4.5, under $100

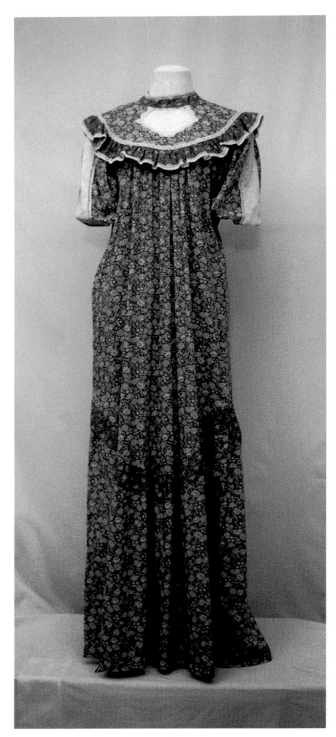

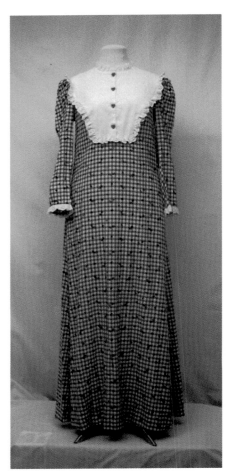

Cotton blend mu`umu`u,
Carol and Mary, 1980s,
97.6.23, under $100

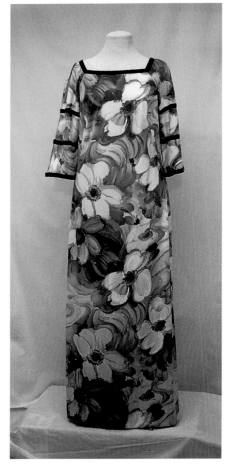

Polyester mu`umu`u,
*Kiyomi Hawaii for Liberty
House,* 1980s, 87.9.7, under
$100

Cotton blend mu`umu`u, *Good Times Hawaii,* 1980s,
TS96.1.36, $100 to $299

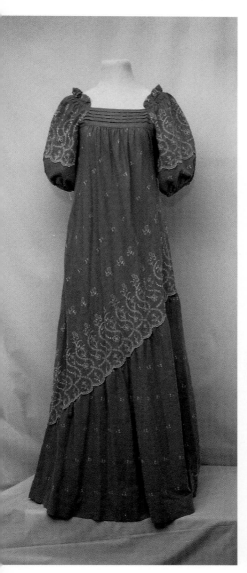

Cotton eyelet mu`umu`u, *Lola Jr. for
Liberty House*, 1980s, 97.6.14, under $100

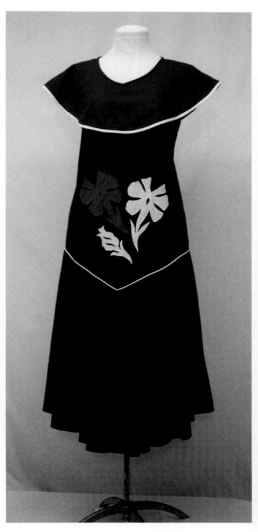

Cotton blend holomu`u, appliqué motif,
courtesy of Lori Chang, 1990s, under $100

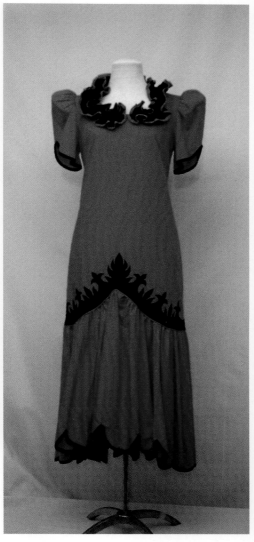

Cotton blend mu`umu`u, Hawaiian quilt
motif appliqué, *courtesy of Lori Chang*,
1990s, $100 to $299

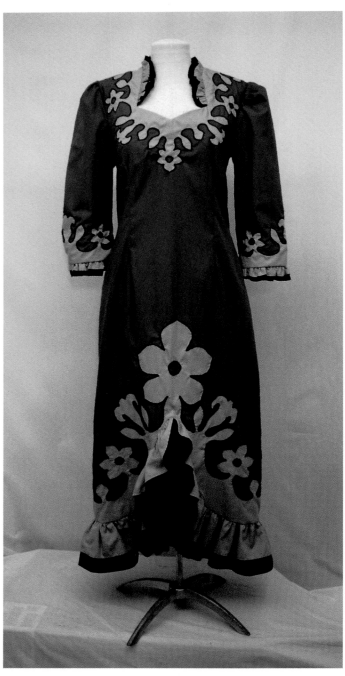

Cotton blend holomu`u, Hawaiian quilt motif appliqué, *Designs by Puamana Crabbe, courtesy of Puamana Crabbe*, 1990s, $300 to $699

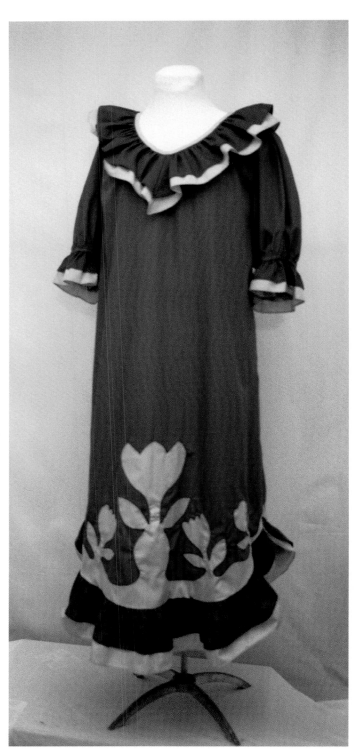

Cotton blend mu`umu`u, Hawaiian quilt motif appliqué, *Designs by Puamana Crabbe, courtesy of Puamana Crabbe*, 1990s, $300 to $699

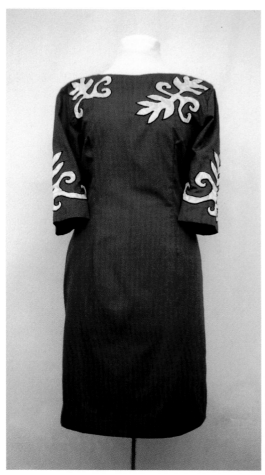

Cotton blend short mu`umu`u, Hawaiian quilt
motif appliqué, *Designs by Puamana Crabbe, courtesy
of Puamana Crabbe,* 1990s, $100 to $299

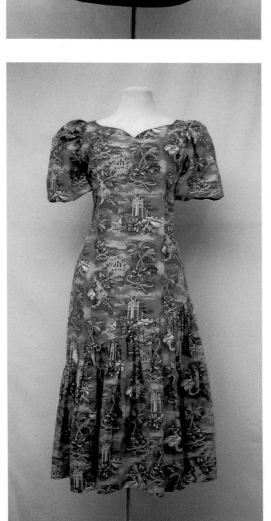

Rayon dress, *Tori Richard, courtesy of Tori Richard,* 1990s, under $100

Cotton blend mu`umu`u, *Reyns,* 1990s,
98.17.8, under $100

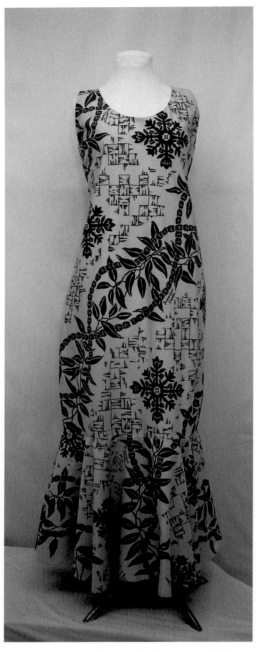

Rayon dress, *Designs by Puamana Crabbe*, *courtesy of Puamana Crabbe*, 1990s, under $100

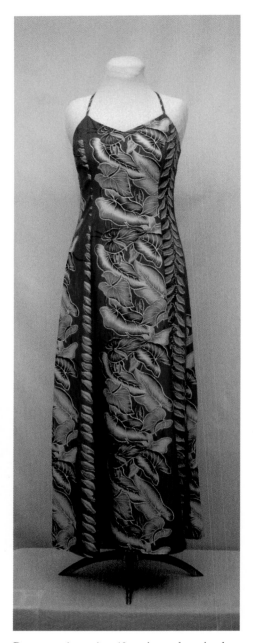

Rayon mu`umu`u, 40s print redone in the 1990s, *Kamehameha, courtesy of Kamehameha Garment Co.*, 1990s, under $100

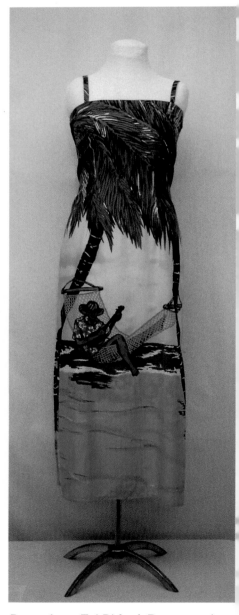

Rayon dress, *Tori Richard*: Dress worn in the 1998 Miss Universe Contest, *courtesy of Tori Richard*, under $100

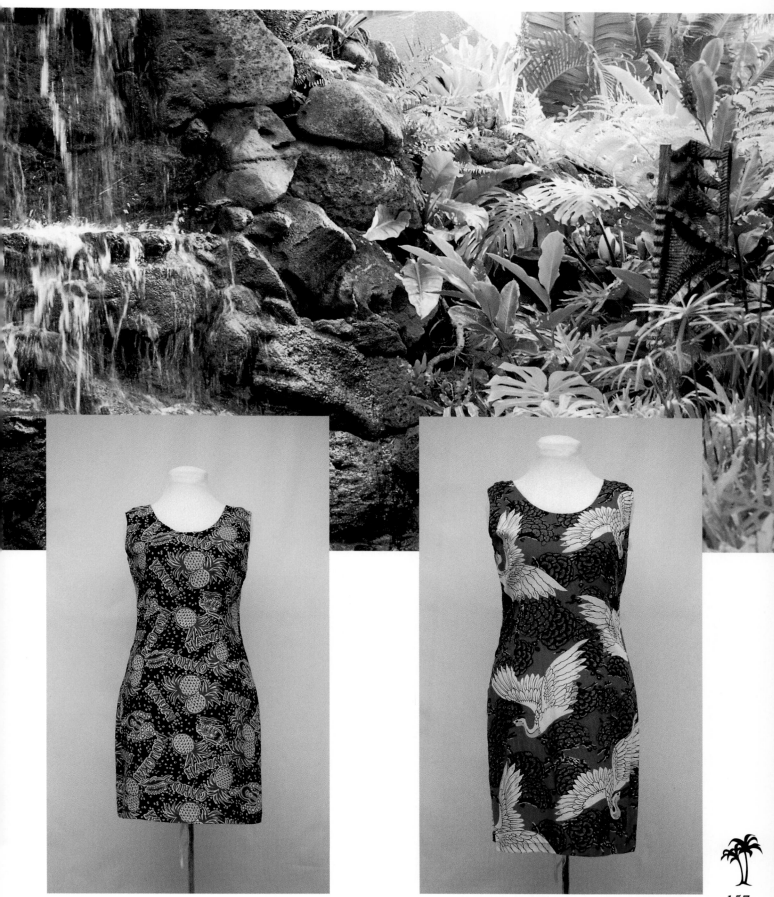

Rayon dress, classic pineapple pattern, *Pineapple Juice,*
courtesy of Pineapple Juice, 1990s, under $100

Rayon dress, *Pineapple Juice, courtesy of Pineapple Juice,*
1990s, under $100

157

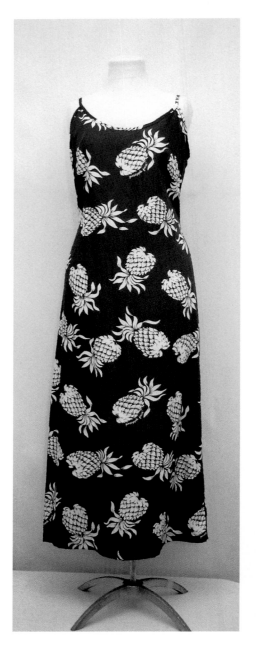

Rayon dress, classic pineapple pattern, *Pineapple Juice, courtesy of Pineapple Juice,* 1990s, under $100

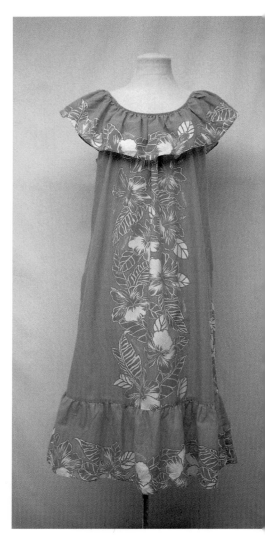

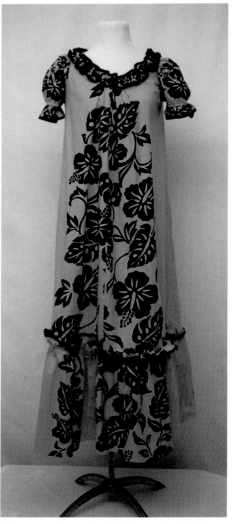

Cotton mu`umu`u, 1990s, under $100

Cotton mu`umu`u, 1990s, under $100

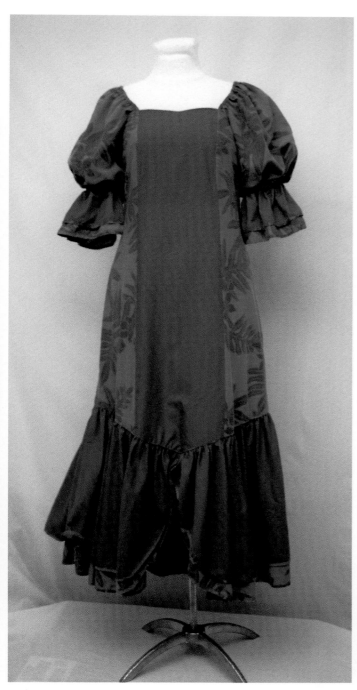

Cotton blend mu`umu`u, *Especially for You*, 1990s, 98.17.6, $100 to $299

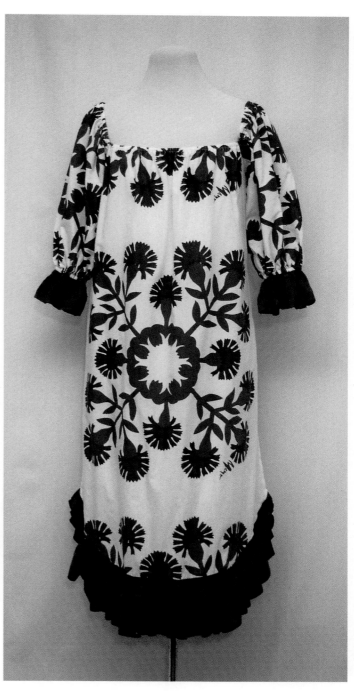

Cotton blend mu`umu`u, *Mamo*, Hawaiian quilt motif appliqué , 1990s, 98.2.2, under $100

159

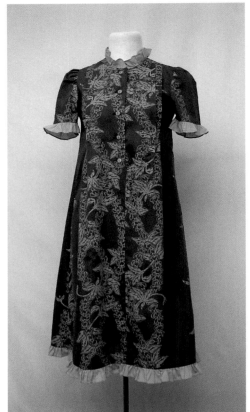

Cotton blend mu`umu`u,
1990s, 98.17.4, under $100

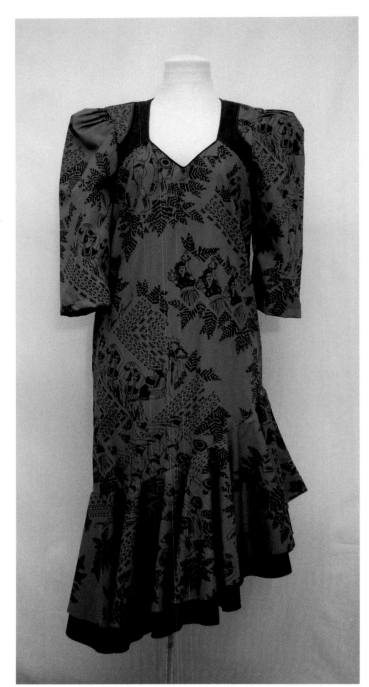

Cotton blend mu`umu`u, *Alan James, courtesy of Alan James,*
1990s, $100 to $299

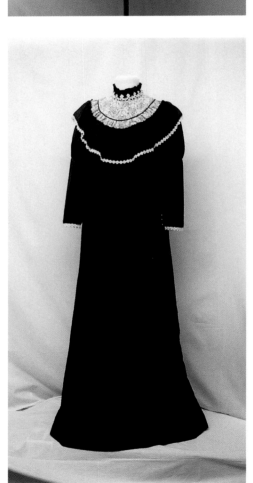

Cotton blend mu`umu`u, *Lola,*
1990s, 95.9.1, under $100

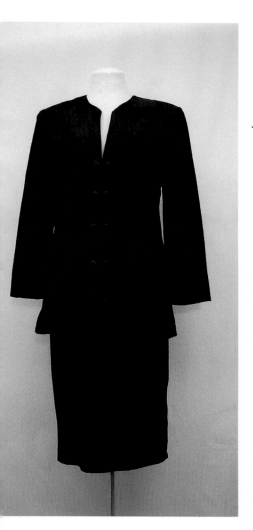

Crepe suit, *Alan James, courtesy of Alan James*, 1990s, $100 to $299

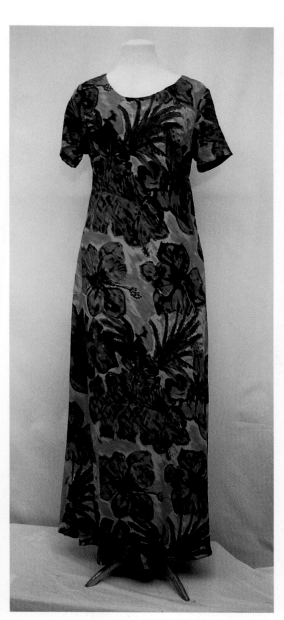

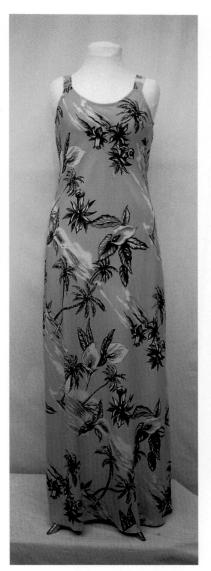

Rayon crepe dress, Hilo Hattie, *courtesy of Hilo Hattie*, 1990s, under $100

Rayon crepe dress, Hilo Hattie, *courtesy of Hilo Hattie*, 1990s, under $100

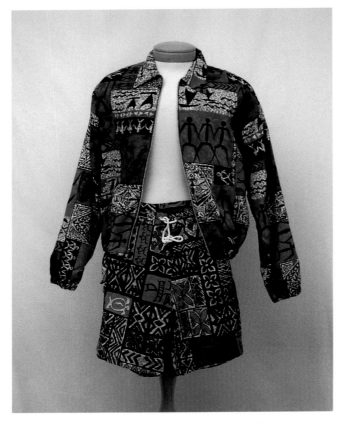

Cotton barkcloth board shorts and jacket, tapa design, *Pineapple Juice*, 1990s, under $100

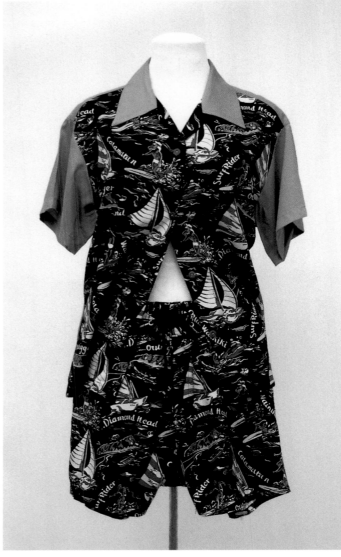

Rayon aloha shirt and shorts, *Pineapple Juice*, *courtesy of Pineapple Juice*, 1990s, under $100

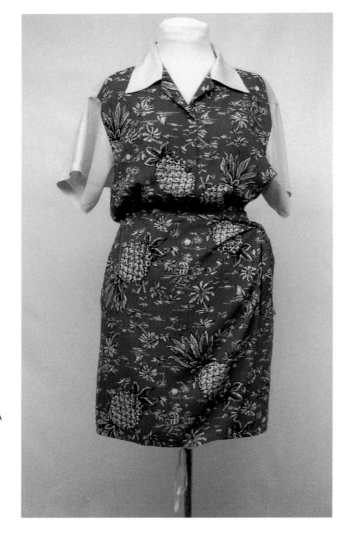

Rayon aloha shirt and sarong skirt, 1990s, *Pineapple Juice*, 1990s, under $100

Men's Wear

      Status is indicated by dress for men as well as women, in Hawai`i. Woe be to the male candidate for a management position who does not know the meanings of dress in Hawai`i. If he comes from the mainland to interview, this candidate is at a disadvantage if he has not studied the dress code and appears with a suit and tie. He must know the importance of the aloha shirt as a business garment, but he must know which kind of shirt is acceptable and the particular styles favored in the company. This is about both sense of place and respect for the culture. As Krauss noted above, Hawai`i has indeed developed a complicated dress code. "The only executives who still wear suits are … lawyers going to court and a few real estate people. I don't even wear a coat and tie to funerals anymore."[92]

      The around-the-clock, all weather uniform for men in Hawai`i is now a crisp, button down aloha shirt with the tails tucked in for business appointments and important social occasions, tails out to be sporty. Such attire is appropriate for any board room, committee meeting, legislative hearing and prac

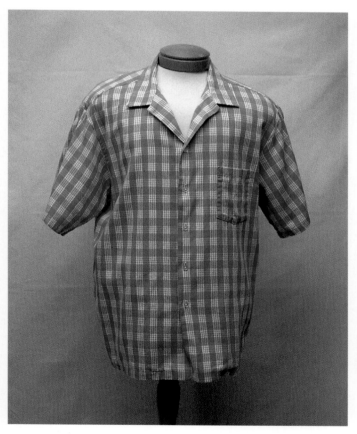

Cotton palaka aloha shirt, *Arakawa's*, 1980s, 98.3.9, under $100

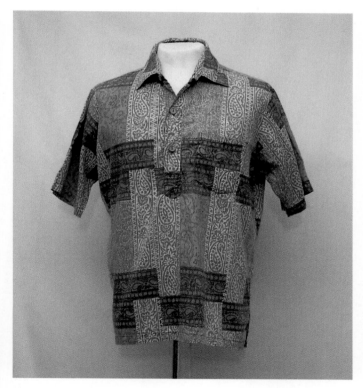

Cotton blend aloha shirt, *Surfline by Liberty House*, 1980s 98.14.9, under $100

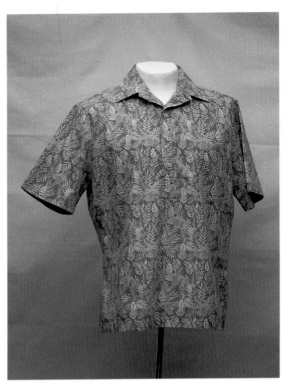

Cotton blend aloha shirt, (identity apparel)
Uniforms by Malia, 1980s, 96.1.17, under $100

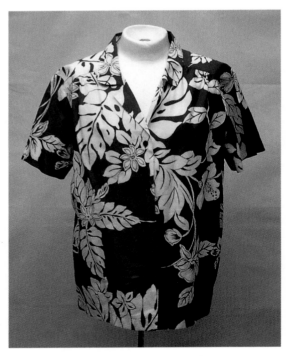

Cotton blend aloha shirt, *Hilo Hattie,* 1980s,
96.1.24, under $100

tically every restaurant in town at any time of the day. But if a male wishes to stand out in such a gathering, if he wishes to subtly one-up his rivals, if he wishes to proclaim his undisputed standing as a native he will wear palaka. To wear palaka is to trade on the snobbery of the Island elite, an exclusive fraternity who call themselves kamaaina, which means children of the land. ... The badge of a male kamaaina is palaka.

For men, aloha shirts are now acceptable fare for nearly every occasion. Some are made of cotton, some are polyester, some are rayon and still others are blends. In any case, the high quality aloha shirt has a pocket that doesn't interrupt the fabric's design, and sometimes buttons that are made out of coconut shells, seeds or bamboo.[93] Fashion reporter Susan Page noted in 1993, "Sales of the shirts are booming. Kramer's Ala Moana store manager Nathan Brovelli, a strapping, handsome local man who looks to be in his 30s, looked a little stunned when I asked him what percentage of his shirt wardrobe was made up of aloha shirts. 'One hundred' was the answer. He said their Cooke Street three button placket pullover style in a light reverse was the big seller. 'Men are wearing brighter colors, hot pinks and purples, that they wouldn't wear five years ago,' Brovelli added."[94]

The 1990s ushered in a new era in aloha attire that relies in part on reproducing the famous prints of the 1940s and 1950s. However, new styles and concepts in Hawaiian prints seem to spring up overnight. The shift is from aloha attire to resort wear with an island feeling.

"It seems the whole world is blooming with prints inspired by our Island style. A recent fashion show in Coeur d'Alene, Idaho, featured the bold and beautiful splashes of color that are uniquely Jams World® stylish men in Milan, Italy, are seen in modish restaurants wearing sophisticated engineered print shirts inspired by - and often made in - Hawai`i. Show-stopper windows at the Las Vegas mega-hotel, the MGM Grand, currently display the latest resort wear from Tori Richard." Josh Feldman [VP at Tori Richard] noted: "The term 'Hawaiian shirt' has come to mean anything that has a bright, colorful, whimsical print on it. The print market on the mainland, in Asia and Europe is explosive. People want to wear a garment they can identify with, just like they used to identify with their favorite slogans on T-shirts. But they can't wear a T-shirt to dinner in a nice restaurant, so they buy a print that relates to their lifestyle."[95]

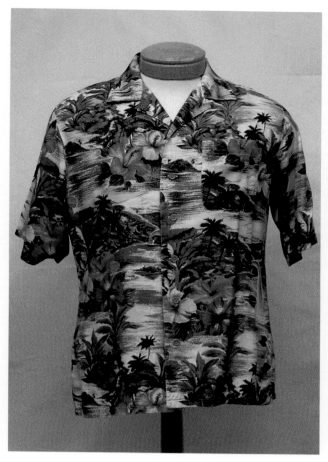

Rayon aloha shirt, *Islander,* 1980s, 97.6.9, under $100

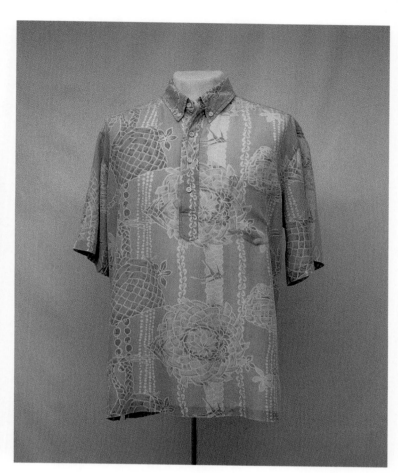

Rayon aloha shirt, *Reyn's,* 1980s, 98.17.50, under $100

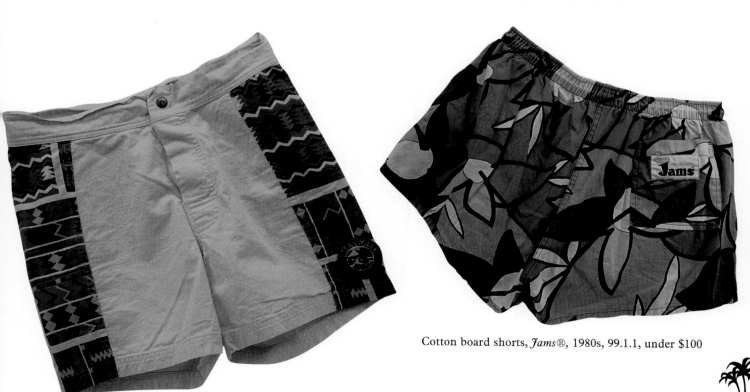

Cotton board shorts, *Jams®,* 1980s, 99.1.1, under $100

Cotton shorts, *Surfline,* 1980s, 99.1.2, under $100

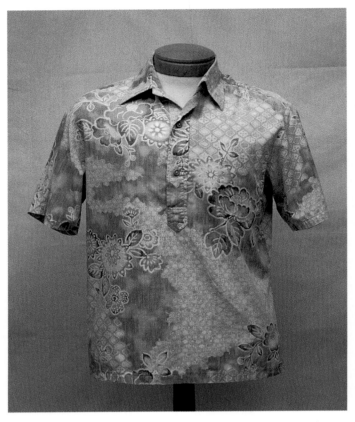

Cotton blend aloha shirt, *Cooke Street*, 1980s, 97.6.5, under $100

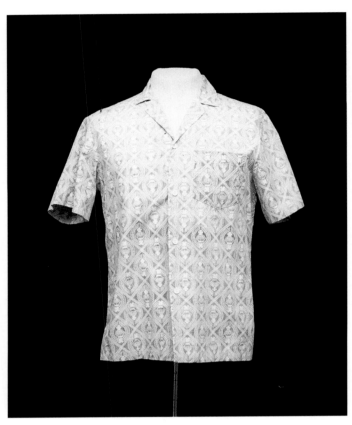

Cotton blend aloha shirt, *Malihini*, 1980s, 98.3.7, 1980s, under $100

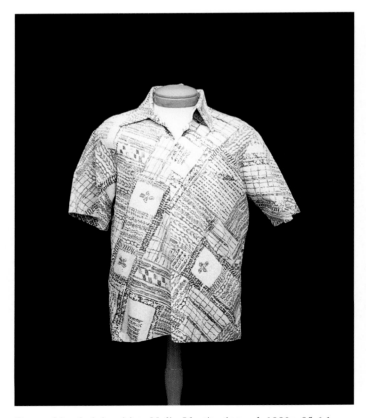

Cotton blend aloha shirt, *Malia Identity Apparel*, 1980s, 95.6.1, under $100

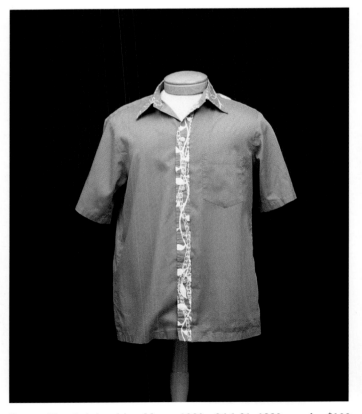

Cotton blend aloha shirt, *Mamo*, 1980s, 96.1.21, 1980s, under $100

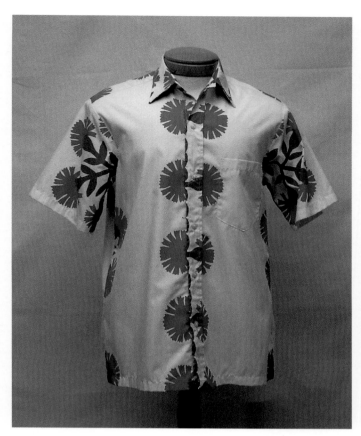

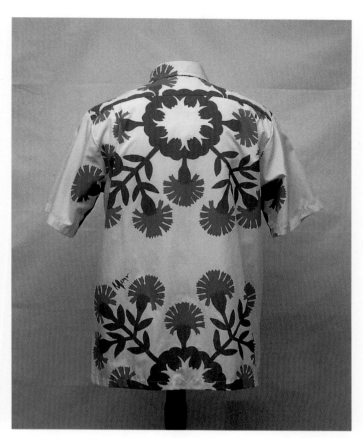

Cotton blend aloha shirt, *Mamo,* 1980s, 97.6.7, under $100

Cotton blend aloha shirt, back view, *Mamo,* 1980s, 97.6.7, under $100

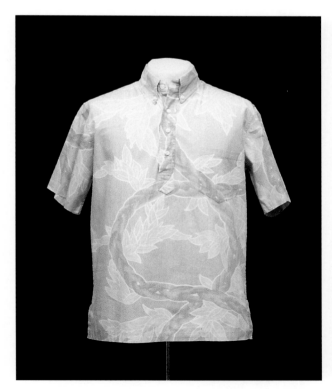

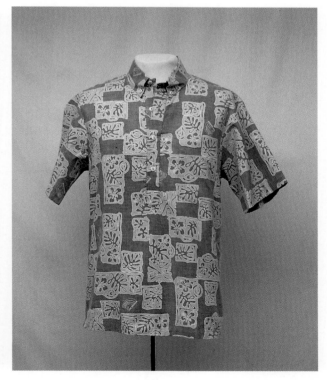

Cotton blend aloha shirt, *Reyn's,* T1980s, TS96.1.1, 1980s, under $100

Cotton blend aloha shirt, *Malihini,* 1990s, 98.17.13, under $100

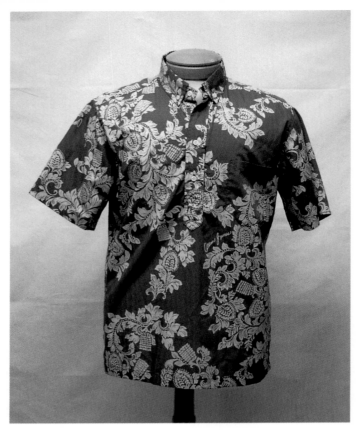

Cotton blend aloha shirt, *Hawaiian Heritage,* 1990s, 98.3.5, under $100

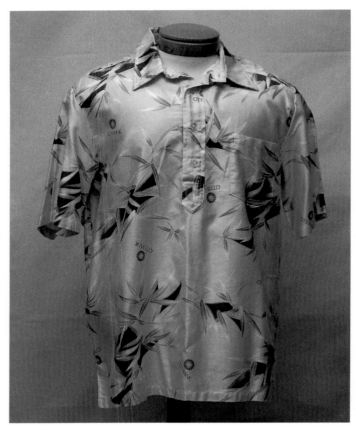

Cotton blend aloha shirt, *High Noon,* 1990s, 96.1.22, under $100

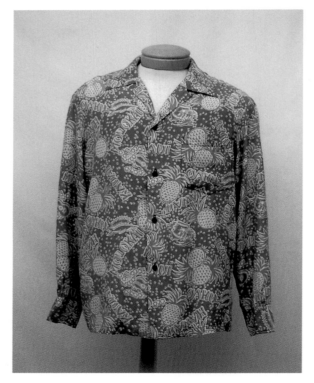

Rayon aloha shirt, *Pineapple Juice,* 98.17.23 1990s, under $100

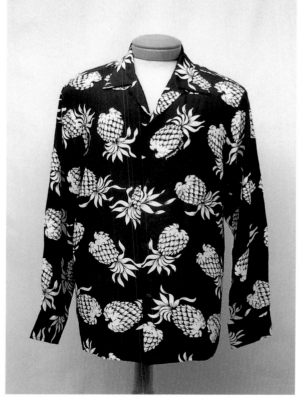

Rayon aloha shirt, *Pineapple Juice ,* 1990s, under $100

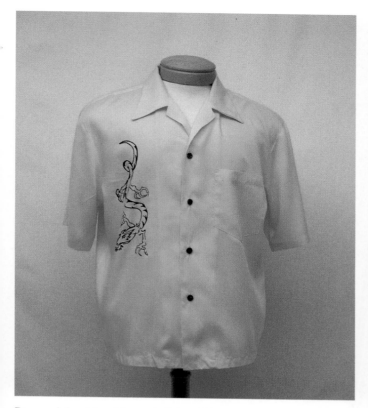

Rayon aloha shirt, *Pineapple Juice*, 1990s, 98.17.21, under $100

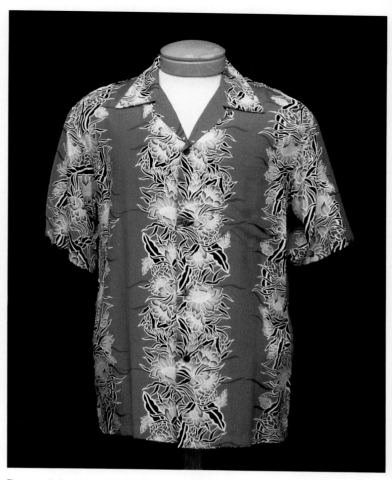

Rayon aloha shirt, *Pineapple Juice*, 1990s, 94.9.2, under $100

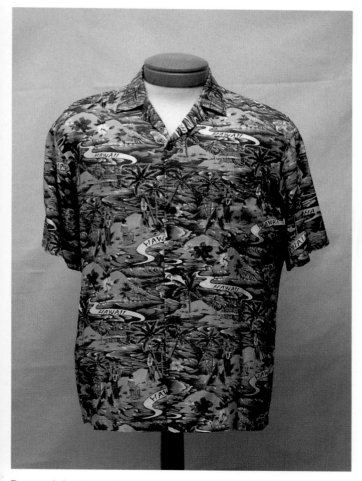

Rayon aloha shirt, *Pineapple Juice*, 1990s, 94.9.1, 1 under $100

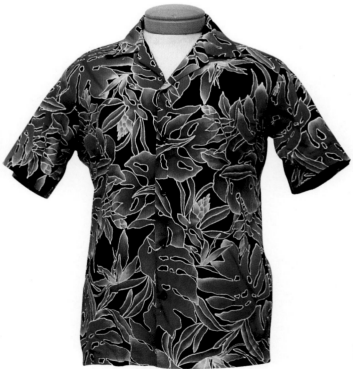

Cotton aloha shirt, *Hilo Hattie*, 1990s, 98.14.2, under $100

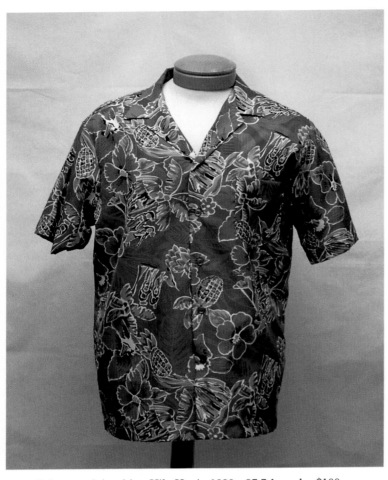

Polyester aloha shirt, *Hilo Hattie*, 1990s, 97.7.1, under $100

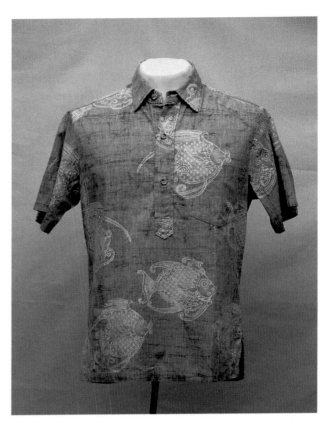

Cotton blend aloha shirt *Kahala*, 1990s, 94.4.3, under $100

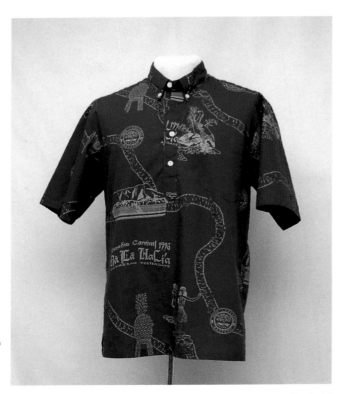

Cotton blend aloha shirt, *Malihini*, 1990s, 98.17.14, under $100

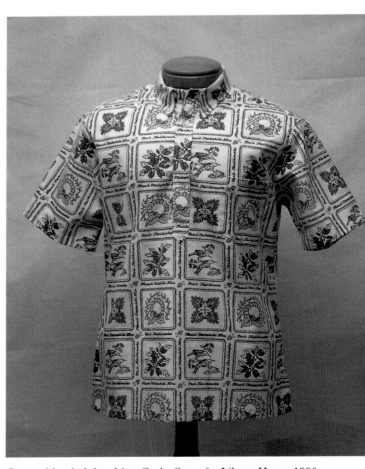

Cotton blend aloha shirt, *Cooke Street for Liberty House*, 1990s , 98.3.2, under $100

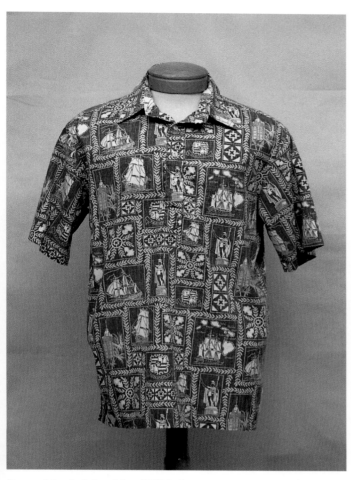

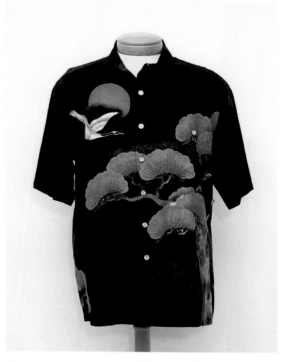

Rayon aloha shirt, *Tori Richard*, *courtesy of Tori Richard*, 1990s, under $100

Cotton blend aloha shirt, *RJC Ltd*, 1990s, 98.3.4, under $100

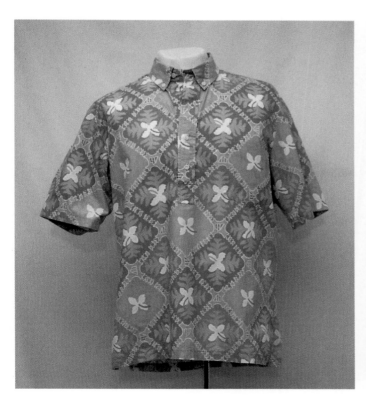

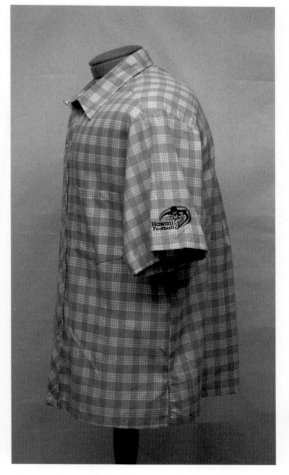

Cotton blend aloha shirt, *Uniforms by Malia*, 1990s, 98.14.11, under $100

Cotton blend palaka shirt, worn by football coaches at the University of Hawai`i (logo on sleeve) *Palaka Hawaii*, 1990s, 95.18.1s, under $100

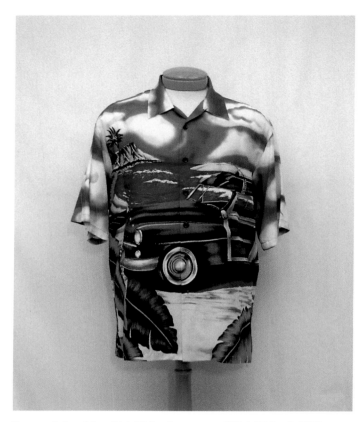

Rayon aloha shirt, *Tori Richard, courtesy of Tori Richard*, 1990s, under $100

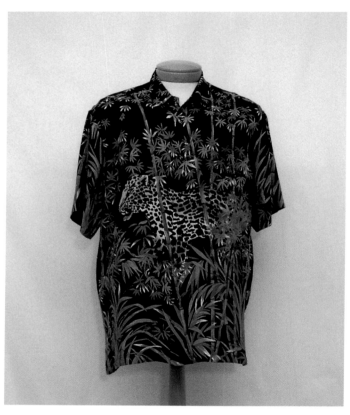

Rayon aloha shirt, *Tori Richard, courtesy of Tori Richard*, 1990s, under $100

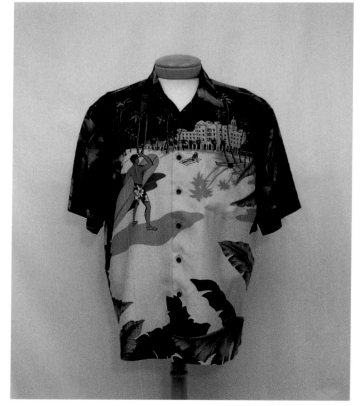

Rayon aloha shirt, *Tori Richard, courtesy of Tori Richard*, 1990s, under $100

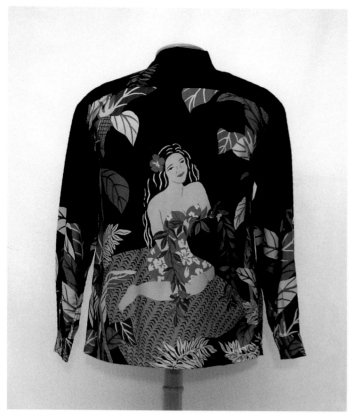

Rayon aloha shirt, *Kamehameha.* 1990s recreation of the 1950s airbrushed shirts, *Courtesy of Kamehameha Garment Co.,* under $100

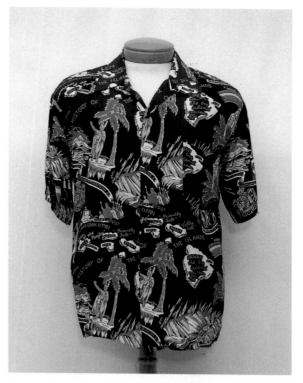

Rayon aloha shirt, *Kamehameha.* 1990s recreation of the 1950s classic silkies, *Courtesy of Kamehameha Garment Co.,* under $100

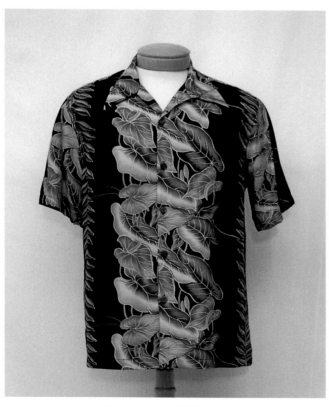

Rayon aloha shirt, *Kamehameha.* 1990s reproduction of *Kamehameha's* famous anthurium print. *Courtesy of Kamehameha Garment Co.,* under $100

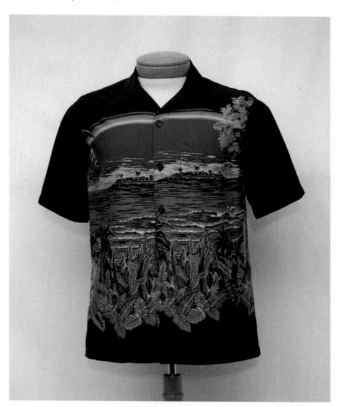

Rayon aloha shirt, *Kamehameha. Courtesy of Kamehameha Garment Co.,* 1990s, under $100

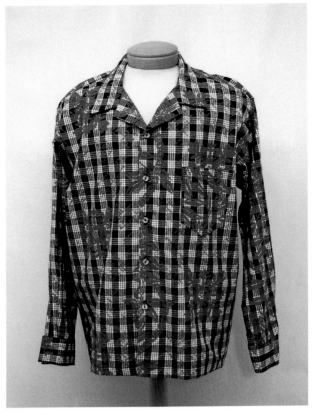

Cotton blend aloha shirt, *Puamana Crabbe;* Hawaiian quilt
motif appliqué, 1990s. *Courtesy of Puamana Crabbe*, under $100

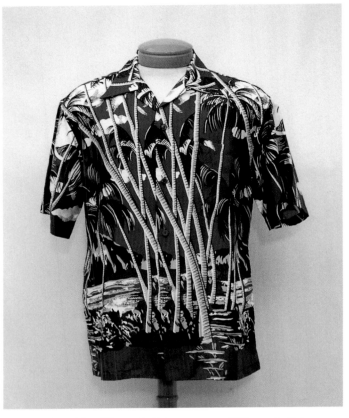

Rayon aloha shirt, *Pineapple Juice, courtesy of Pineapple Juice*,
1990s, under $100

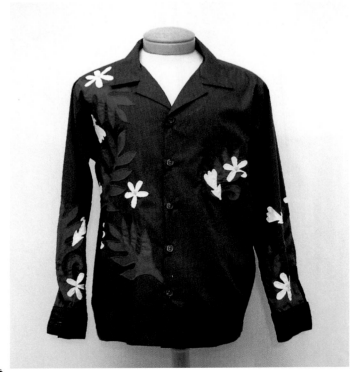

Palaka aloha shirt, *Puamana Crabbe*, Hawaiian motif screen
printed over palaka, 1990s. *Courtesy of Puamana Crabbe*,
$100 to $299

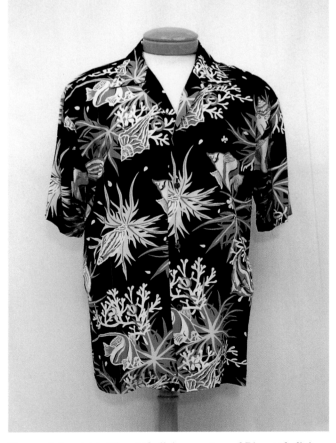

Rayon aloha shirt, *Pineapple Juice, courtesy of Pineapple Juice*,
1990s, under $100

10. Accessories

The Wearing of the Lei

Throughout the long history of ancient Hawai`i, before people from the Western world came to the Islands, Hawaiians wore garlands of flowers and shells around the head or shoulders. Traditionally, the head and shoulders were considered to be sacred parts of the body. Today, lei are symbolic of Hawai`i, and are fragrant garlands of flowers worn either around the neck, head, or on a hat. In the Boat Days (1890 through the 1930s) the custom of giving lei to arriving and departing steamship passengers began. Many passengers, on passing Diamond Head on their return to the US mainland, would throw their lei into the water. This practice is incorrectly explained as a legend — that it was believed that if the lei arrived on shore, the passenger would return to the Hawaiian Islands one day.[96] (In reality, however, this tradition was created in the 1920s to prevent people from throwing lei back onto the docks and creating a mess to be cleaned up.) This 'legend' was publicized by the Matson Lines, as well as the Hawai`i Tourist Bureau.[97]

A lei is given along with a kiss of aloha; the gift of a lei symbolizes respect, honor, and love. The consummate gift of aloha is a lei, bestowed on a person with a kiss. Lei are given on birthdays, graduations, anniversaries and other important occasions; they are special gifts. Marie McDonald, a lei specialist, notes that "many people have difficulty saying 'I love you.' In Hawai`i, we get around the words by giving a lei."[98]

The custom of wearing leis was made famous in the early twentieth century when tourists arriving by ship would be greeted with lei on their arrival into the Islands. Even today, lei sellers continue to produce leis for tourist arrivals at the airport. Available at florist shops and lei shops throughout the islands, leis are generally displayed in long colorful strands, tied upon purchase for the consumer.

There are several different kinds of lei, and they can be made of shells, paper, candy, ribbon, fabric, currency and even golf balls. However, the most common kind of lei that are worn as accessories to aloha attire are made of either shells (as in the Ni'ihau lei) or flowers, the subject of this section. Each kind of floral lei has a different look, smell, and sometimes, meaning. Plumeria blossoms are very fragrant, and are commonly found in lei. Dendrobium and vanda orchids are also frequently used in lei – they are durable, lasting longer than other lei. There is protocol with regard to lei, depending on the occasion. A bride generally wears a white jasmine or pikake lei, and a bridegroom wears the maile lei open at both ends.

While most lei are worn in a long strand, circling the neck and shoulders (the lei umauna) there are other styles as well. A shorter lei, worn like a choker around the neck is called the lei ai. Lei worn around

Lei for sale

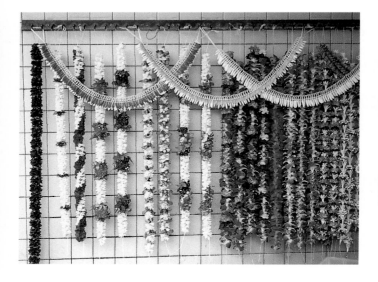

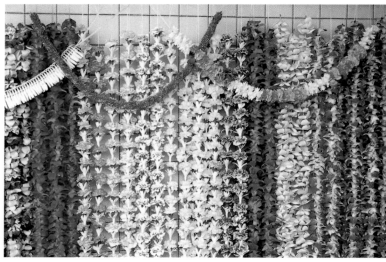

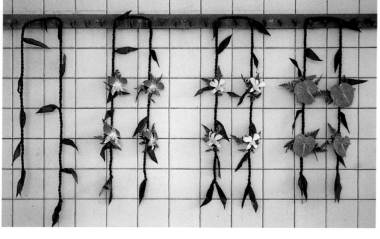

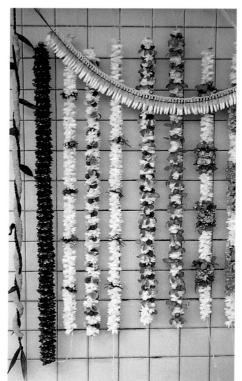

the head are lei po'o. Yet other lei are worn over the shoulders, and not tied together. The ends hang loose. These are lei made of green leaves, the maile and ti leaf lei. The ti leaf lei are made by twisting the leaf into a rope-like strand, leaving the tip projecting outward when a new leaf is added to the strand. The maile lei is rare and considered the finest of all lei.[99]

Each island has a particular lei associated with it; Maui, "The Valley Isle," is known for the lokelani (rose) lei, while the favored lei of Kauai, "The Garden Isle" is the green mokihana. O'ahu, "The Gathering Place" has the gold 'ilima lei as its favorite lei. The Big Island (Hawai`i), also known as "The Orchid Isle," has the `ohi`a a lehua made of feathery red and yellow blossoms. Moloka'i, "The Friendly Isle," has a green lei of kukui (candlenut) leaves and nuts. Lana'i, "The Secluded Isle," has a feathery yellow vine called kauna'oa kahakai. Kaho'olawe, "The Barren Isle," has a teal blue lei of hinahina ku kahokai (heliotrope). Ni'ihau, "The Kapu Isle," is well known for its Ni'ihau shell lei. These lei made of pupu shells are made in long, and very valuable, strands.[100]

176

Jewelry

Before westerners arrived in the Hawaiian Islands, people of both sexes wore necklaces and garlands of shells, nuts and flowers. This practice has continued unabated to the present time. Jewelry made in the Islands may be constructed of a variety of local materials. Lauhala weaving is used for bracelets and even rings (see below). Traditionally, most jewelry has been made in the form of necklaces of shells and seeds. In spite of the association of necklaces with femininity in the Western world, Hawaiian men have comfortably worn necklaces of shells and nuts, though the length of the strands are generally shorter for men than those worn by women.

Hawaiian heirloom jewelry is very popular in Hawai`i today; it is modeled after jewelry given by Queen Victoria of England to Hawaii's Queen Liliuokalani in 1887. Hawaiian heritage jewelry is done in gold; designs of Hawaiian flowers and plants often dominate the design. Usually, the bangle bracelets have contrasting lettering done in black, using an Old English script. Generally, Hawaiian names are used on the bracelets, and Hawaiian words or phrases are engraved in it as well.

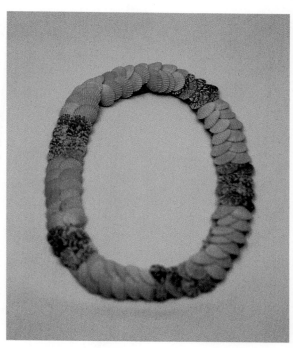

Shell hatband, 1930s, 98.13.12, $700 to $999

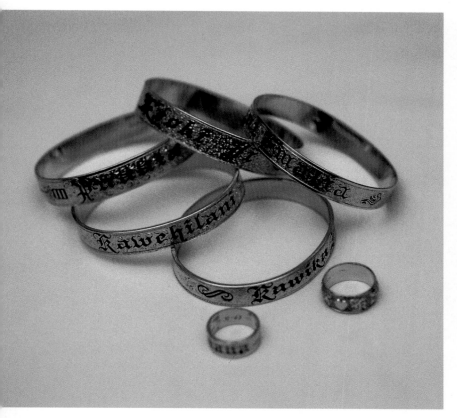

Hawaiian Heirloom jewelry, *Courtesy of Ginny Baker*, $1,000+

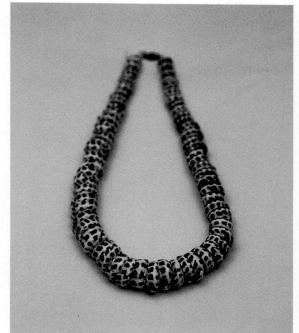

Tiger shell necklace from Maui. 1950s, 98.13.18, $300 to $699

177

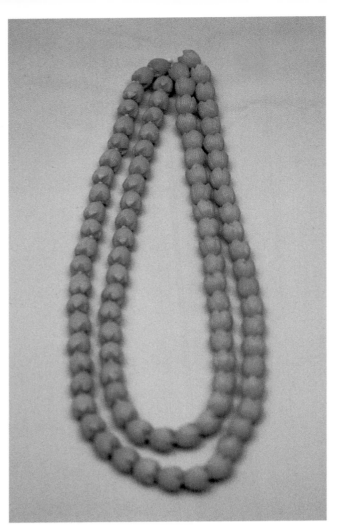

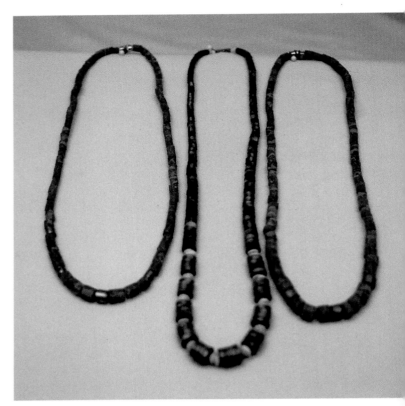

Coral necklaces, 1980s, 98.13.14, $100 to $299

Pikake necklace of ivory, gift received by Bernadine Barrow aboard the *Lurline* in 1951, 98.13.13, $300 to $699

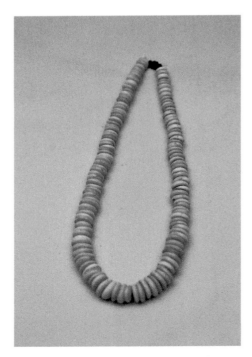

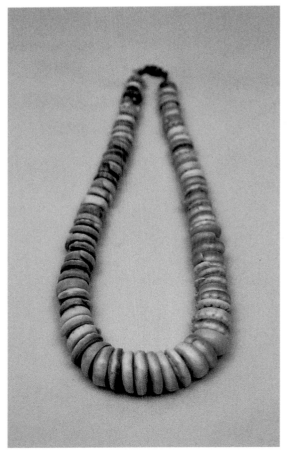

Puka shell necklace worn by men, 1950s, 98. 13.17, under $100

Puka shell necklace worn by men, 1950s, 98. 13.16, $100 to $299

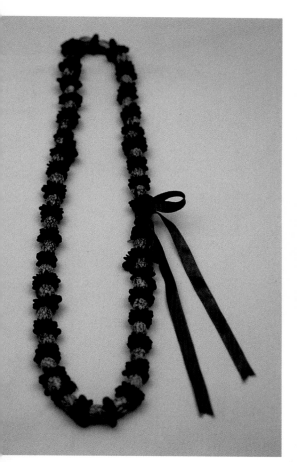

Seed lei, *courtesy of Barbara Harger*, under $100

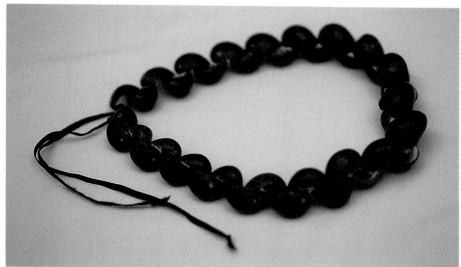

Kikui nut lei, *courtesy of Barbara Harger*, under $100

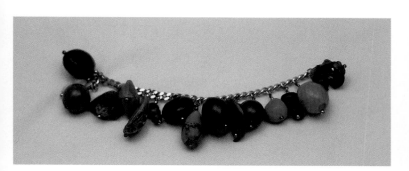

Bracelet of varied Hawaiian nuts, 1950s, 98.16.2, under $100

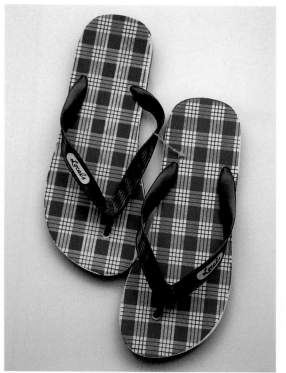

Rubber slippers, *Locals*, 1990s, under $100

179

Lauhala Hats and Accessories

For centuries, lauhala (woven from the leaf of the hala tree) has been woven in Hawai`i for use in mats, hats, fans, purses, and jewelry. Traditionally, the most authentic kama`aina-style lauhala hats were woven by the older ladies in Kona (on the Big Island).

There was a time when one could identify a local male by the style of his hat woven from the limber and durable fronds of the hala tree. There were cowboy hats from the cool, grassy plateau of Waimea on the Big Island. There were fishermen's hats from the parched and sunny seashore of Kailua, Kona. There were wide-brimmed planter's hats, smart Panama hats, and everyday hats for people who worked in the cane fields.[101]

The demand for lauhaha hats kept native weavers very busy until the past two decades. Unfortunately, lauhala hats became rare for a while, as few lauhala weavers continued to produce hats in the 1980s. While most lauhala weavers have been women, one of the best lauhala hat makers today is a man living on Oahu, in Honolulu.[102] Fortunately, lauhala weaving is seeing a resurgence in Hawai`i, with outstanding artists emerging, especially on the Big Island. Ka Ulu Lauhala O Kona is an organization dedicated to the perpetuation of lauhala weaving, and this group is determined to preserve this ancient Hawaiian craft.[103]

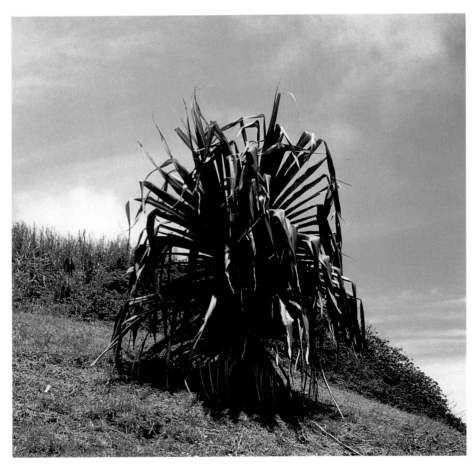

Hala tree — the leaves from the Hala tree are used to weave lauhala mats, hats and other accessories

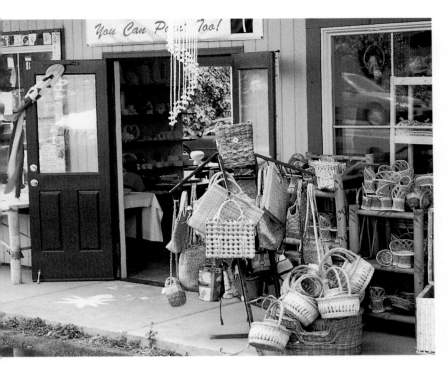

Kauai shop with lauhala accessories and mats

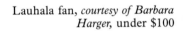

Lauhala fan, *courtesy of Barbara Harger,* under $100

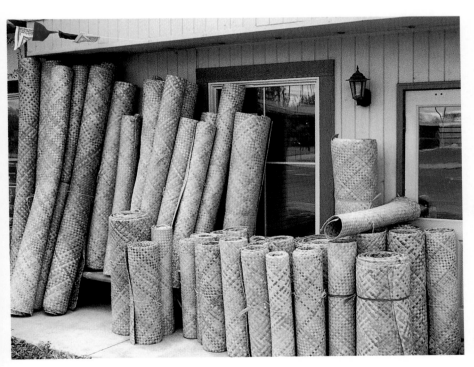

Lauhala mats for sale at a shop on Kauai.

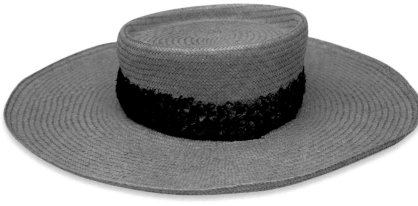

Lauhala hat with band of peacock
feathers, 1980s , 98.13.10, $300 to $699

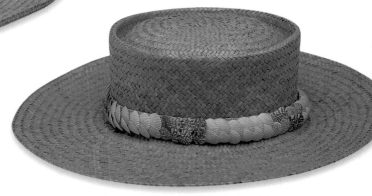

Lauhala hat from 1950s with band from
1930s of shells, 98.13.12, $700 to $999

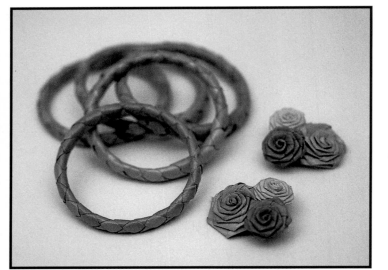

Lauhala bracelets and earrings,
courtesy of Ginny Baker, $100 to $299

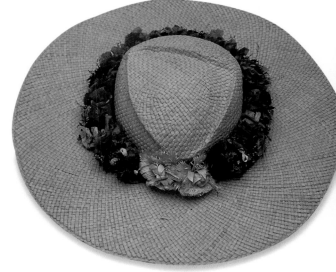

1950s Lauhala hat *"Caddy, original
Hawaiian Lauhala Hat – Honolulu"* with
band of haku lei, 99.10.1, $100 to $299

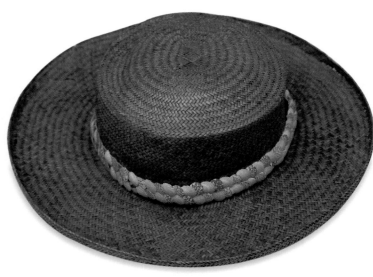

1950s lauhala hat worn on plantation, with shell
band from the 1930s, 98.13.11, $700 to $999

11. Labels & Values

Numerous factors are used in determining values on vintage garments. It is important to understand that vintage clothing is subject to fads, just like contemporary fashion. The following remarks concern the key determinants of value in the late 1990s while the trend has favored "silkies" from the post World War II era. Fabric is critical; rayon garments are more valuable than other fabrics. Patterns are also very important in determining values on Hawaiian garments, and though just as many Asian designs have been produced in aloha attire, Hawaiian motifs are favored by collectors; hence they draw higher prices. Similarly, aloha shirts bring higher prices than clothing produced exclusively for women. The more spectacular colors and patterns draw the highest prices. Condition, era, size, and label (especially those made in Hawai`i) are also important considerations in determining values for vintage Hawaiian clothing.

Placing values on vintage clothing is difficult, as no two items are the same. At the same time, regional markets are wildly different in terms of the prices that garments will fetch. Japan is usually the most expensive market for aloha attire, followed by Hawai`i. To even things out, in determining value for garments in this book I have used prices one would find in Hawai`i. I have leveled the playing field by having appraisals done with an assumption that all garments are in excellent condition and in desirable sizes.

The labels in the following pages are from the garments seen in the preceding pages. Most come from major manufacturers from the Hawaiian Garment Industry. They are arranged alphabetically in the pages that follow, and the labels of each manufacturer are arranged in approximate chronological order.

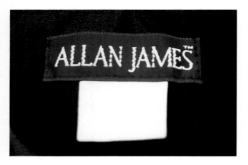

Alan James

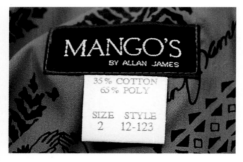

Mangos/ Alan James

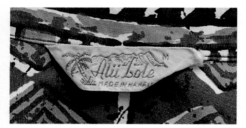

Alii Lode

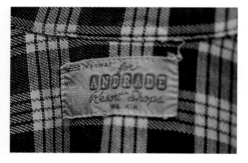

Andrade Resort Shops

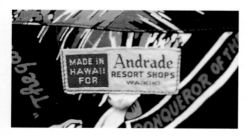

Made in Hawaii for Andrade Resort Shops

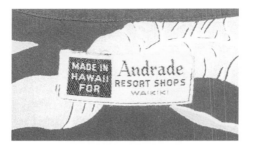

Made in Hawaii for Andrade Resort Shops

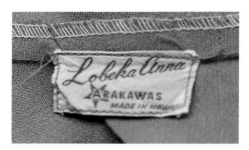

Lobeka Anna Arakawa's Made in Hawaii

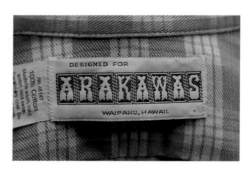

Designed for Arakawa's, Waipahu, Hawaii

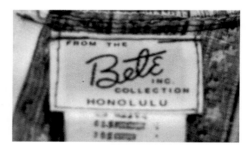

From the Bete, Inc. Collection, Honolulu

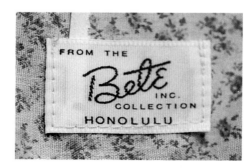

From the Bete, Inc. Collection, Honolulu

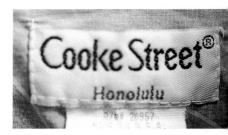

Cooke Street, Honolulu (Cooke Street is a Tori Richard label)

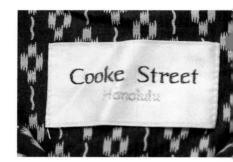

Cooke Street, Honolulu

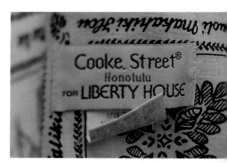

Cooke Street, Honolulu for Liberty House

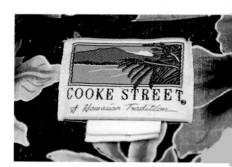

Cooke Street, a Hawaiian Tradition

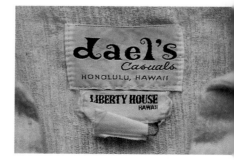

Dael's Casuals, Honolulu

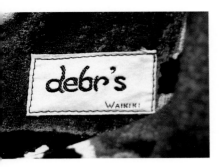

Debr's, Waikiki

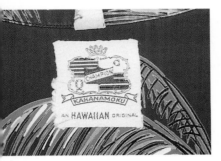

Champion Duke Kahanamoku, An Hawaiian Original

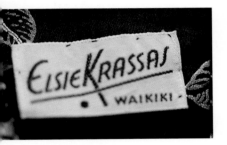

Elsie Krassas, Wakiki

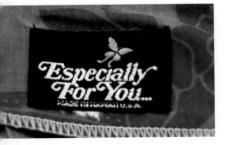

Especially for You

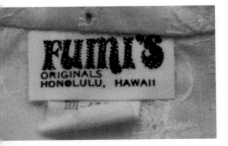

Fumi's Originals, Honolulu, Hawaii

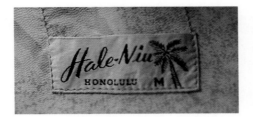

Hale Niu, Waikiki

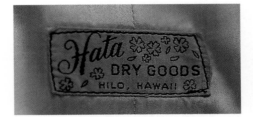

Hata Dry Goods, Hilo Hawaii

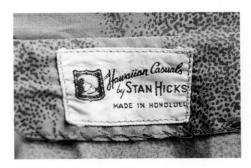

Hawaiian Casuals by Stan Hicks, Made in Honolulu

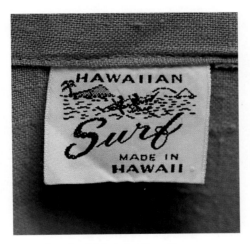

Hawaiian Surf, Made in Hawaii

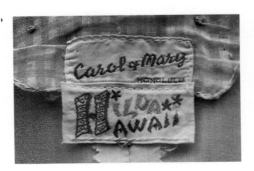

Hilda Hawaii, Carol and Mary, Honolulu

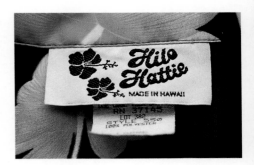

Hilo Hattie, Made in Hawaii

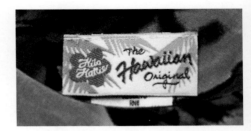

Hilo Hattie, the Hawaiian Original

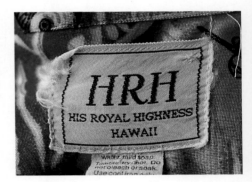

HRH His Royal Highness

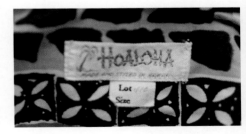

HoAloha, Made and Styled in Hawaii

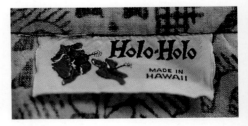

Holo Holo, Made in Hawaii

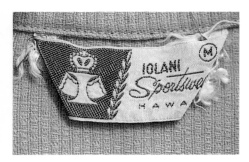

*Iolani Sportswear, Hawaii Queen Surf,
100% Cotton*

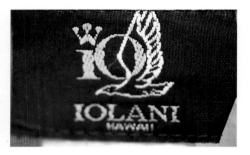

Iolani Hawaii

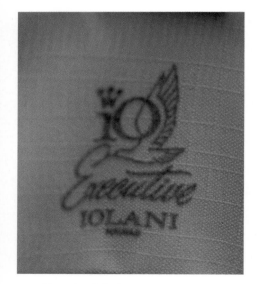

Executive Iolani

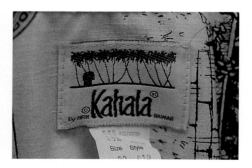

Kahala

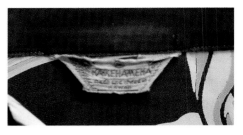

Kamehameha, Made and Styled in Hawaii

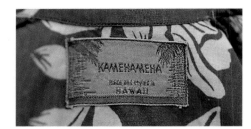

Kamehameha, Made and Styled in Hawaii

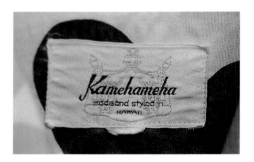

Kamehameha, Made and Styled in Hawaii

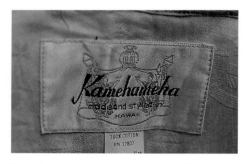

Kamehameha, Made and Styled in Hawaii

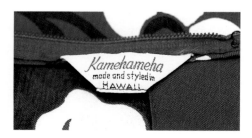

Kamehameha, Made and Styled in Hawaii

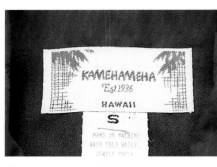

Kamehameha, est. 1936

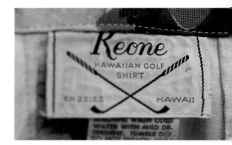

Keone Hawaiian Golf Shirt

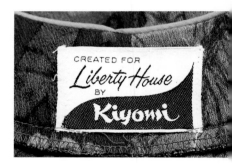

Created for Liberty House by Kiyomi

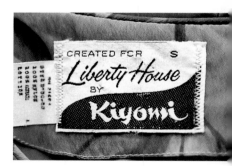

Created for Liberty House by Kiyomi

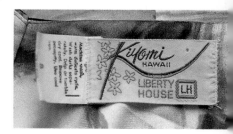

Kiyomi of Hawaii Liberty House

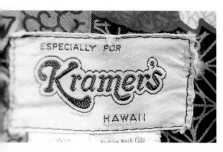

Especially for Kramers, Hawaii

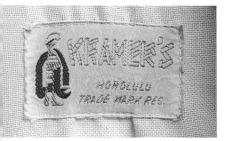

Kramer's, Honolulu

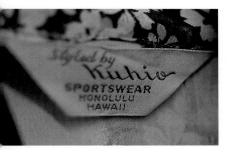

Styled by Kuhio Sportswear, Honolulu Hawaii

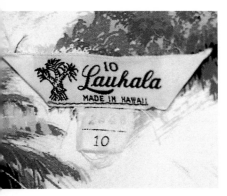

Lauhala

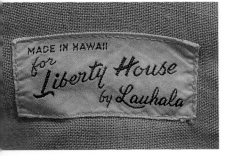

Made in Hawaii for Liberty House by Lauhala

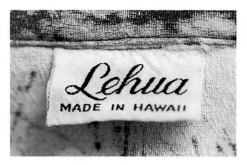

Lehua, Made in Hawaii

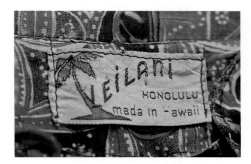

Leilani Honolulu, Made in Hawaii

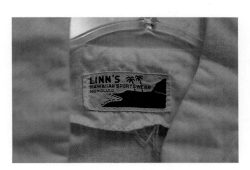

Linn's Hawaiian Sportswear, Honolulu

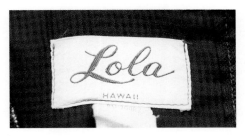

Lola Hawaii

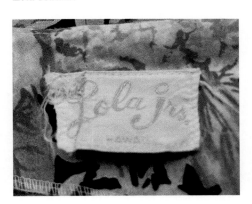

Lola Jr. Hawaii

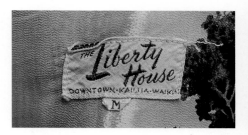

Liberty House

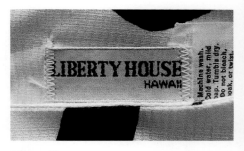

Liberty House

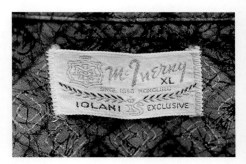

McInerny, Iolani Exclusive

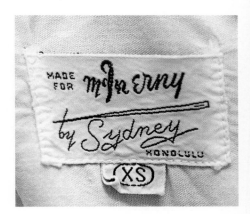

McInerny, by Sydney

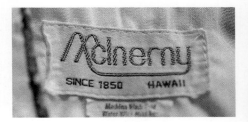

McInerny, since 1850 Hawaii

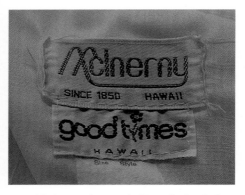

McInerny, since 1850 Hawaii, Good Times

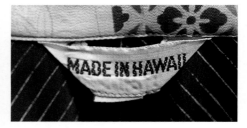

Made in Hawaii

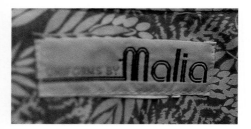

Uniforms by Malia

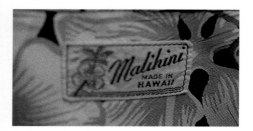

Malihini, Made in Hawaii

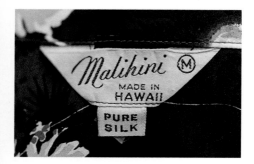

Malihini, Made in Hawaii

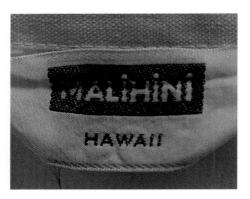

Malihini, Hawaii

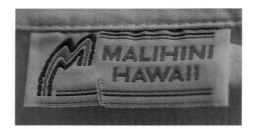

Malihini, Hawaii

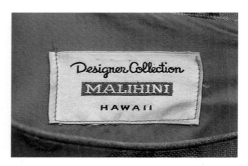

Designer Collection, Malihini, Hawaii

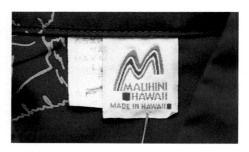

Malihini, Hawaii

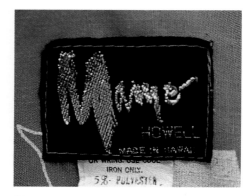

Mamo

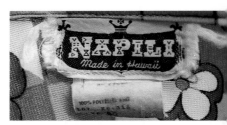

Napili, Made in Hawaii

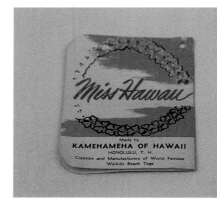

Miss Hawaii, Kamehameha of Hawaii

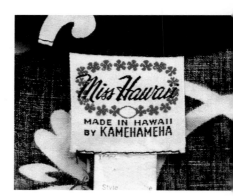

Miss Hawaii, Made in Hawaii by Kamehameha

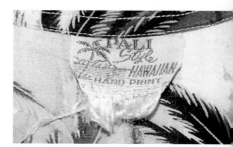

Pali Style Hawaiian

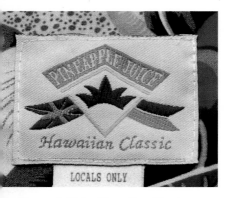

Pineapple Juice Hawaiian Classic

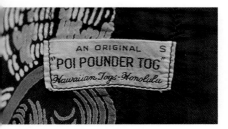

Original Poi Pounder Tog, Hawaiian Togs Honolulu

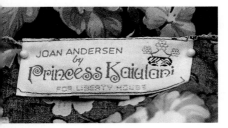

Joan Andersen by Princess Kaiulani for Liberty House

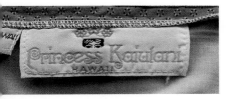

Princess Kaiulani Hawaii

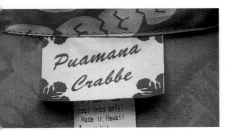

Puamana Crabbe

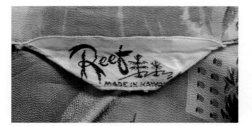

Reef, Made in Hawaii

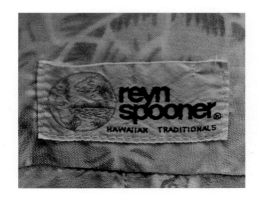

Reyn Spooner Hawaiian Traditionals

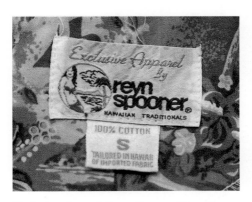

Exclusive Apparel Reyn Spooner Hawaiian Traditionals

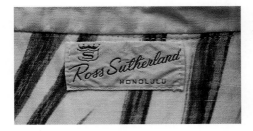

Ross Sutherland, Honolulu

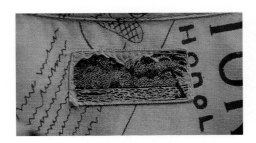

Royal Hawaiian Quality Garments

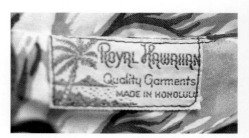

Royal Hawaiian Quality Garments Made in Honolulu

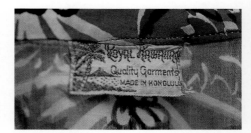

Royal Hawaiian Quality Garments Made in Honolulu

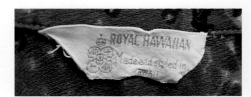

Royal Hawaiian Made and Styled in Hawaii

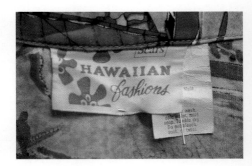

Sears Hawaiian Fashions

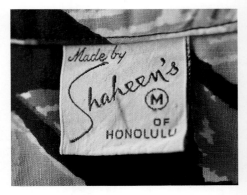

Shaheen's of Honolulu

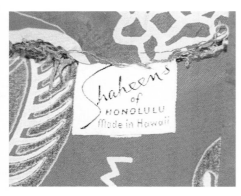

Shaheen's of Honolulu, Made in Hawaii

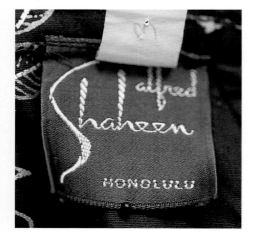

Alfred Shaheen, Honolulu

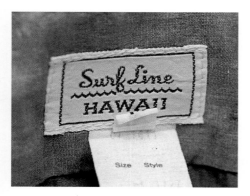

SurfLine Hawaii

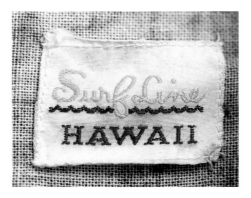

SurfLine Hawaii

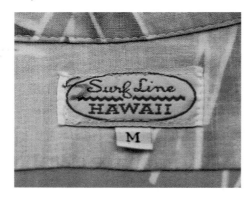

SurfLine Hawaii

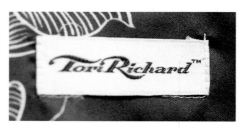

Tori Richard

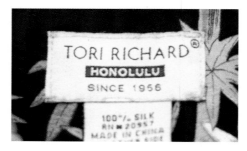

Tori Richard Honolulu, Since 1956

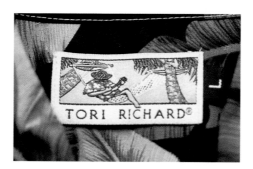

Tori Richard

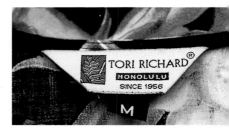

Tori Richard Honolulu, Since 1956

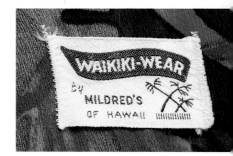

Wakiki Wear by Mildred's of Hawaii

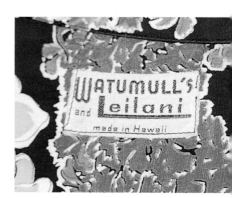

Watumull's and Leilani, Made in Hawaii

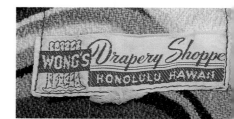

Wong's Drapery Shoppe, Honolulu, Hawaii

Notes

1 Mark Twain, *New York Tribune*, 1973. Reprinted in *Paradise of the Pacific* V.75, January 1963, pp. 13-15.

2 Curtis Manchester, Aloha Attire: A Geographic Perspective. *AAG Conference Handbook*. 1999.

3 Dress is a term that includes clothing, grooming and accessories — which are especially important in Hawai'i.

4 Miss A. J. Allen, *Dr. White's Travels and Oregon Adventures*, (1836: reprint, Ithaka, NY: Andrus, Gauntlet, 1850); C. Barnard, *Voyage Around the World* (London: J. Lindon, 1829); von Kotzebue, O. (1821) *Kotezebue's voyage of discovery 1815-1818*. London: Longman, Thirst, Rees, Orme and Brown. Tyreman, J & Bennett, G. (1831). *Journal of voyages and travel*. London: Fredrick Westley and A.H. Davis."Voyage"; Tyreman and Bennett, "Journal"; Barbara. Lyons, "The First Holoku." *Hawai`i Historical Review*. (1963): 54-55.

5 Otto von Kotzebue, *Voyage*; Maria Chamberlain to James Patton, 25 September 1820, Missionary letters, Hawai'i Mission Children's Society Library, Mission Houses Museum, Honolulu, HI; Lucy G. Thurston, *Life and Times of Mrs. Lucy G. Thurston, Wife of Rev. Asa Thurston, Pioneer Missionary to the Sandwich Islands, Gathered from Letters and Journals Extending Over a Period of More Than Fifty Years, Selected and Arranged by Herself* (Ann Arbor, MI: S.C. Andrews, 1882); Gail Stewart, "Ancient Hawaiian Dress and the Influence of European Dress on it 1778-1820," (Master's thesis, Univ. of Hawai'i at Manoa, 1977).

6 von Kotzebue, *Voyage*.

7 "Holoku — Origin and Evolution," *Picturesque Honolulu*, (Honolulu: Hawaiian Gazettte, 1907): 44-45; Edwin McClellan, "Holoku and Muumuu," *Forecast Magazine*, (Honolulu: Outrigger Canoe Club, 1950): 12; Lucy Thurston, *Life and Times*.

8 Lucy Thurston, *Life and Times*; Loomis, *Grapes of Caanan*; Emma Fundaburke, *The Garment Manufacturing Industry of Hawai'i*. (Honolulu: Economic Research Center, 1965); "Holoku"; McClellan, "Holoku and Muumuu," 12.

9 Emma Fundaburke, *Garment Manufacturing Industry of Hawai'i*, 1965; Gloria Furer, "Designs of Hawaiian Wear," *Proceedings of the American Association of College Professors of Textiles and Clothing* (1983): 13.

10 Mary Anderson, *Scenes in the Hawaiian Islands and California*,(Boston: American Tract Society,1865); Helvenston, "Mother Hubbard."

11 Patricia Grimshaw, *Paths of Duty: American Missionary Wives in Nineteenth Century Hawai'i* (Honolulu: University of Hawai'i Press, 1989).

12 Herb Kawainui Kane. The Shirt That Shouts Aloha! *Islands*. 29-35.

13 Linda Arthur, "Cultural Authentication Refined: The Case of the Hawaiian Holoku," *Clothing and Textiles Research Journal*, 15, 3(1997): 129-139.

14 "Holoku".

15 *Sales Builder*. July 1940, p. 3-14.

16 Chris Oliver. Buddhism in Hawai'i Dates to 1889. *Honolulu Advertiser*. 5/2/99, G-3.

17 The largest ethnic groups in Hawai'i are Caucasian (22%), Japanese (20%), Hawaiian and part-Hawaiian (21%), Mixed race non-Hawaiians, (21%), Filipino (10%) and Chinese (5%).Hawai'i State Data Book, 1996.

18 DeSoto Brown, *Hawai'i Recalls*. Honolulu. Editions Limited. 1982, p. 10-11, 98.

19 Emma Fundaburke, *Development of Apparel Manufacturing, Textile Designing &Textile Printing in Hawai'i*. 1965.

20 Fashion History Made With Aloha. *Fashion Sports Hawai'i*. 1991. Honolulu Pub.Co.

21 Barbara Kawakami. 1993. *Japanese Immigrant Clothing in Hawai'i 1885-1941*. Honolulu. University of Hawai'i Press P. 147.

22 "Holoku", 1907.

23 Barbara Kawakami.

24 Ibid.

25 Interview with Goro Arakawa, *Honolulu Star Bulletin*, June 16, 1964.

26 Honolulu Star Bulletin, June 16,1964

27 Thomas Steele. 1984. *The Hawaiian Shirt*.

28 DeSoto Brown. *Hawai'i Recalls*, Honolulu.Editions Limited. 1982.

29 Alfred Shaheen, Interview, 2/1/99.

30 DeSoto Brown and Gunter Von Hamm, interviews. Fall 1998.

31 Most of ads reporting fabric available in stores referred to yardage for home sewing. Gump's was a store that dealt only with home interiors, not yardage for sewing. Their ads mentioning tropical prints referred to fabric for draperies, slipcovers and upholstery.

32 *Sales Builder*, No. 7, Vol. 13. July 1940, p. 13.

33 Sparkey Doo. Interview, 9/98.

34 Cleo Evans, *Honolulu Advertiser*, 1/22/61.

35 Lorna Arlen, Pins and Needles in Hawaii: Honolulu's Newest Industry- Manufacturing Women's Clothes- Has Grown

in the Last Two Years to Million Dollar Proportions. *The Honolulu Advertiser*. 2/19/39.

36 Barbara Laughlin, *Hawaiian Garment Companies.* unpublished manuscript.

37 Unfortunately, the shirt made famous in the film "From Here to Eternity" has been incorrectly dated in other books as a result of confusion over the licensing of Duke's name. Duke Kahanamoku licensed his name three times; it was not until the second time that Duke's name was connected to the famous "Here to Eternity" shirt – this was 1950. Publicity photos of the release of Duke Kahanamoku shirts on the mainland, printed in the New York Post and the Daily Compass in January 1950 clearly date this shirt to 1950. Yet another line of swimwear, much like the original 1939 garments, were produced by Kahala in 1961 under a third agreement.

38 Watumull's Buys Garment Firm. *Honolulu Star Bulletin*, 4/13/55.

39 Cleo Evans.

40 Sparkey Doo, Interview 11/10/98; Alfred Shaheen,Interview 2/1/99.

41 Ibid.

42 Jonathan Moor, Hawaiian Punch, *Gentlemen's Quarterly* Summer 1978

43 Mun Kin Wong, Interview 11/10/98.

44 John Heckathorn. 1996. *Honolulu Magazine*, August. p. 52-55

45 Ibid.

46 Phyllis Tortora and Billie Collier, 1997, *Understanding Textiles*, Prentice Hall.

47 Marty Wentzel, The Shirt that Says Aloha. *Pleasant Hawaii*. 1989. 30-57; Alfred Shaheen, Interview 2/1/99.

48 Fundaburke, 1965, 305.

49 Alfred Shaheen.

50 Emma Funderburke, 1965, p.37.

51 Putting Hawaiian Fashion on the Map. *Honolulu Star Bulletin*, 9/7/80.

52 Blake Green, 101 Uses For Aloha Attire. *San Francisco Chronicle*, 9/14/85. P. 13.

53 Alfred Shaheen.

54 Sales Builder, No. 7, Vol. 13. July 1940, p. 13.

55 Alfred Shaheen.

56 Alfred Shaheen.

57 DeSoto Brown, p. 110; Alfred Shaheen.

58 DeSoto Brown, Bishop Museum Archivist. *Daily Compass,* 1/23/1950; *New York Post,* 1/18/1950.

59 Women's Wear Daily, Thursday, 1/18/1950.

60 Alfred Shaheen.

61 Wentzel, the Shirt that Says Aloha, p. 57.

62 Alfred Shaheen.

63 DeSoto Brown, Interview, 6/6/99; Nancy Schiffer,

Hawaiian Shirt Designs. Schiffer Publications. 1997; p. 38.

64 Dee Dickson. Hawaii, Fashions As Colorful As The Islands. *Aloha Magazine.* 1979.

65 Alfred Shaheen.

66 Carol Pregill, President of Hawaii Fashion Industry Association. Interview 1999.

67 Herb Kawainui Kane.

68 DeSoto Brown, Interview, 6/6/99.

69 Dee Dickson.

70 Honolulu Star Bulletin, October 8,1961. P. 27

71 Alfred Shaheen.

72 Heckathorn.

73 Barbara Laughlin. 1998.

74 Ibid.

75 Andrew Gomes. Uniforms Sustaining Life of Aloha Wear Manufacturers. *Pacific Business News.* 9/7/98.

76 Dee Dickson.

77 Andrew Gomes.

78 C. Sinnex. A Pattern for Success. *Midweek.* 6/29/94.

79 DeSoto Brown.

80 Andrew Gomes.

81 Hawaiian Rights and Sovereignty. Available: http:www.hookele.com/kuhikuhi/ea.html

82 Andrew Gomes.

83 Rath, Paula. *Honolulu Advertiser.* 10/14/97, pp. C1-3.

84 Ed Rampell, Hawaiiana Manufacturers Find Gold Out West. *Pacific Business News.* 5/7/99.

85 Terry Shipley (VP Sales, Pomare) in Blake Green, 101 Usies for Aloha Attire, *San Francisco Chronicle,* 9/14/85.

86 Carol Pregill.

87 Andrew Gomes.

88 Andrew Gomes.

89 Bob Krauss. Our Hawaii: *The Best Of Bob Krauss.* Island Heritage Publishing. 1990.

90 Bob Krauss.

91 Carol Pregill.

92 Bob Krauss.

93 Wenzel.

94 Susan Page, 1993, *Midweek,* 5/12/93.

95 Rath, Paula. *Honolulu Advertiser.* 10/14/97, pp. C1-3.

96 Laurie Shimizu Ide, *Hawaiian Lei Making.* 1998. Honolulu. Mutual Publishing.

97 DeSoto Brown, Interview, 6/6/99.

98 Marie McDonald, *Ka Lei.*

99 Ibid.

100 Laurie Shimizu Ide.

101 Bob Krauss.

102 Bob Krauss.

103 Paula Rath, Hats: Art of Lauhala Weaving Revived. *Honolulu Advertiser,* C1-3, 6